WEALTH OF HEALTH

WEALTH OF HEALTH

Prince Akubue
Foreword by Prof Josephat O Ogbuagu

ISBN 13: 9781543021868
ISBN-10: 1543021867
Library of Congress Control Number: 2017908031
CreateSpace Independent Publishing Platform
North Charleston, South Carolina

DEDICATION

This Handbook is dedicated to the Almighty God for His love and infinite mercies.

ACKNOWLEDGEMENTS

THIS ACCOMPLISHED GREAT and unique work is a synergistic product of experience and many great minds. I am forever grateful to the inspiration and wisdom of great men and women who supported this work.

I must acknowledge as well the many friends, colleagues, students and teachers who assisted, advised, and supported this writing effort over the years. I need to express my gratitude and deep appreciation to true friends who have consistently helped keep perspective on what is important in life and shown how to deal with reality.

My amiable appreciation to my spouse, Mrs. Akubue Prince Peace Ifeome for her endearing countenance.

I express my immense appreciation to all who directly or indirectly contributed to the success of this book.

CONTENTS

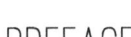

PREFACE

THIS BOOK OF Wealth of Health is for the enlightenment of the entire human race irrespective of class, custom and culture. It shows how to cope with health and lifestyle issues. But it does more to probe beneath the surface of lifestyle and points to the real meaning and reasons behind current health challenges, risks and life-threatening conditions.

The inspiration for this book arose from the desire to enlighten and instill a greater appreciation in society at large, the conception and perception of healthy living lifestyle and to inspire modern folks to explore its fascinating chapters.

However, it is educating and invaluable materials for everyone. It discusses about alcohol abuse and misuse, diet and nutrition, drug abuse and misuse, exercise effects, skin care and sunscreen protection, coping with stress, toothache and mouth odour, mood disorders and how to overcome a host of health challenges and risks.

The author has meticulously gathered the pieces together for us to build a healthy life. It is simply a unique and exquisite text with copious and explicit explanations.

FOREWORD

This "Wealth of Health" is a gift that carries in it the awesome power to shape our lifestyle and wellbeing. The reality of a healthy lifestyle and wellbeing is far more rewarding once the unfortunate and distressing images of health risks and poor health are dispelled.

This book is both revealing and rewarding as the author has captured and conveyed what works and what does not work in our drive to stay healthily fit. It is a recommended companion to Nutritionists, Dietetics, Physicians, gym Instructors, Psychologists, Psychiatrists, Dermatologists and host of other professionals and non-professionals. The in-depth analysis and discussions on health matters are captivating.

Healthy lifestyle must not just be a slogan, it must be a responsible concern that is put into practice to lower lifestyle diseases and health risks. As we journey into the second decade of the new millennium, the challenges to good health and wellbeing are great tasks that need our attention.

Prof Josephat Ogbuagu, *mni*
Provost, Federal College of Education Technical Umunze, Nigeria

C H A P T E R   1

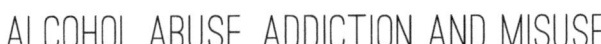

ALCOHOL ABUSE, ADDICTION AND MISUSE

1.1. DEFINITION OF ALCOHOLIC BEVERAGES

AN ALCOHOLIC BEVERAGE is a drink that typically contains 3% – 40% alcohol (ethanol). Alcoholic beverages are divided into three classes: beers, wines, and spirits (distilled beverages). They are legally consumed in most countries around the world. More than 100 countries have laws regulating their production, sale, and consumption.

1.2. ALCOHOL CONCENTRATION (ABV)

Typical ABV ranges	
Beers	3–15%
Wines	8–17%
Fortified wines	15–22%
Spirits	15–98%
Fruit juices	< 0.1%
Cider, wine coolers	4–8%

The concentration of alcohol in a beverage is usually stated as the percentage of alcohol by volume (ABV, the number of ml of pure ethanol in 100 ml of beverage) or as proof. In the United States, proof is twice the percentage of alcohol by volume at 60 degrees Fahrenheit (e.g. 80 proof = 40% ABV). Degrees proof were formerly used in the

United Kingdom, where 100 degrees proof was equivalent to 57.1% ABV. Historically, this was the most dilute spirit that would sustain the combustion of gunpowder.

Ordinary distillation cannot produce alcohol of more than 95.6% ABV (191.2 proof) because at that point alcohol is an azeotrope with water. A spirit which contains a very high level of alcohol and does not contain any added flavoring is commonly called a neutral spirit. Generally, any distilled alcoholic beverage of 170 proof or higher is considered to be a neutral spirit. Most yeast cannot reproduce when the concentration of alcohol is higher than about 18%, so that is the practical limit for the strength of fermented beverages such as wine, beer, and sake. However, some strains of yeast have been developed that can reproduce in solutions of up to 25% ABV.

1.3 TYPES OF ALCOHOLIC OR FERMENTED BEVERAGES

The variety of alcohol types, different brands, and mixing ingredients is sometimes overwhelming.

Wine

Fermentation with the stems, seeds, and skins of the grapes will increase the tannin content of the wine.

Wine is a fermented beverage produced from grapes. Wine involves a longer fermentation process than beer and also a long aging process (months or years), resulting in an alcohol content of 9%–16% ABV. Sparkling wine can be made by means of a secondary fermentation.

Beverages called "fruit wines" are made from fruits such as plums, cherries, or apples. The kind of fruit must be specified on the label.

Beer

Beer is a beverage fermented from grain mash. It is made from barley or a blend of several grains. If the fermented mash is distilled, then the beverage is a spirit. Beer is the most consumed alcoholic beverage in the world.

2

Cider

Cider or cyder is a fermented alcoholic beverage made from any fruit juice; apple juice (traditional and most common), peaches, pears ("Perry" cider) or other fruit. Cider alcohol content varies from 1.2% ABV to 8.5% or more in traditional English ciders. In some regions, cider may be called "apple wine".

1.4. HEALTH RISKS OF ALCOHOLIC BEVERAGE ABUSE AND MISUSE

"Good health!" Yet, paradoxically, millions of people worldwide are drinking themselves into the grave.

Alcohol misuse is a multifaceted problem that includes hazardous use, harmful use, and dependence. Hazardous use, as defined by the World Health Organization, is "a pattern of alcohol consumption carrying with it a risk of harmful consequences," physical, mental, or social. It includes drinking more than the limits recommended by health authorities or imposed by the law. Harmful use, also called alcohol abuse, involves drinking that which is already provoking either physical or mental damage but has not yet led to dependence. Dependence has been described as "the loss of control to abstain from drinking." An alcohol-dependent person craves alcohol, continues to drink despite various alcohol-induced problems, and suffers from withdrawal in its absence.

No matter what your age, gender, race or nationality, you are not free from the risks of hazardous drinking. Just what does alcohol do to the body? What are the health dangers of overdrinking? What is generally considered a safe level of alcohol consumption? And why boozing?

Dangerous for the Mind

Ethanol, the chemical compound present in most alcoholic drinks, is a neurotoxin—that is, a substance that can damage or destroy the nervous system. Someone who is drunk is, in fact, suffering from a form of poisoning. In large quantities, ethanol causes coma and death. For instance, among students in Japan, the practice of ikkinomi, or alcohol chugging, causes deaths every year. The body is able to convert ethanol into harmless substances, but this is not accomplished immediately. If alcohol is consumed at a faster rate than the body can handle it, ethanol builds up in the system and begins to interfere noticeably with brain function. In what way?

Speech, vision, coordination, thought, and behavior are all connected with an incredibly complex series of chemical reactions in the brain's neurons, or key cells. The presence of ethanol modifies those reactions, suppressing or enhancing the role of certain neurotransmitters—chemicals that relay signals from neuron to neuron. The stream of information in the brain is thus altered, preventing the brain from functioning normally. That is why when a person drinks too much, he or she develops slurred speech, blurred vision, sluggish movement, and weakened behavioral restraints and inhibitions—all common symptoms of intoxication.

With prolonged exposure to alcohol, brain chemistry adapts to counter the poisonous effect of ethanol and to maintain normal nerve function. This leads to tolerance, whereby the same amount of alcohol has less of an effect than it would have had previously. Dependence occurs when the brain has adapted so much to the presence of alcohol that it cannot operate properly without it. The body craves alcohol to maintain the chemical balance. When a person is deprived of alcohol, his brain chemistry is totally destabilized and withdrawal symptoms, such as anxiety, trembling, or even seizures, set in.

Besides causing modifications of brain chemistry, alcohol abuse can lead to cell atrophy and destruction, altering the brain's very structure. While partial recovery is possible with abstinence, some of this damage seems to be irreversible, further affecting memory and other cognitive functions. Damage to the brain is not just the result of long-term exposure to alcohol. Research seems to indicate that even relatively short periods of alcohol abuse can be harmful.

Liver Disease and Cancer

The liver plays a vital role in metabolizing food, combating infection, regulating blood flow, and removing toxic substances, including alcohol, from the body. Prolonged exposure to alcohol damages the liver in three stages. During the first stage, the breaking down of ethanol slows the digestion of fats, causing them to build up in the liver. This is called steatohepatitis, or fatty liver. In time, chronic inflammation of the liver, or hepatitis, sets in. While alcohol can cause hepatitis directly, it also appears to lower the body's resistance to hepatitis B and hepatitis C viruses. If unchecked, inflammation causes cells to burst and die. Compounding this damage, alcohol seems to trigger the natural system of programmed cell death called apoptosis.

The final stage is cirrhosis. The vicious cycle of continuous inflammation and cell destruction causes irreversible scarring. Eventually, the liver becomes lumpy, instead of remaining spongy. Finally, scar tissue prevents blood from flowing normally, leading to liver failure and death.

Alcohol's effect on the liver has another insidious side effect—the liver is less capable of playing its defensive role in counteracting the effect of cancer-forming agents. In addition to favoring the development of cancer of the liver, alcohol greatly increases the risk of cancer of the mouth, the pharynx, the larynx, and the esophagus. What is more, alcohol makes the mucous membranes in the mouth more easily penetrated by cancerous substances in tobacco, elevating the risk for smokers. Women who drink daily are at greater risk of breast cancer. According to one study, the risk for those who drank three or more alcoholic beverages per day was 69 percent higher than that of nondrinkers.

Poisoned Babies

A particularly tragic outcome of alcohol abuse is its effect on the unborn. "Alcohol is far worse for the developing fetus than any other abused drug," reports the International Herald Tribune. When a pregnant woman drinks, her developing child also drinks, and the toxic effect of alcohol is especially devastating at this formative stage of the fetus. Alcohol causes irreversible damage to its central nervous system. Neurons do not form properly. Cells are killed off. Other cells end up located in the wrong place.

The result, fetal alcohol syndrome (FAS), is the foremost cause of mental retardation in newborns. Difficulties encountered by FAS children include intellectual impairment, language problems, developmental delay, behavioral dysfunction or deficit, slow growth, hyperactivity, and hearing and sight disorders. Many FAS babies are also born with characteristic facial deformities.

In addition, children whose mothers drank even moderate amounts of alcohol during pregnancy can suffer from certain disabilities, including behavioral problems and learning deficits. "You don't have to be an alcoholic to hurt your baby," remarks Professor Ann Streissguth, of the fetal alcohol and drug unit at the University of Washington, "you just have to be drinking enough and pregnant." The report of the French National Institute of Health and Medical Research Alcool—Effets sur la santé notes: "The absorption of alcohol is deleterious during the whole gestational period, and no minimal dose has ever been established below which there are no risks." Consequently, the wisest course for women who are pregnant or planning a pregnancy may be not to drink any alcohol at all.

Safe Drinking
The list of health risks mentioned above is by no means exhaustive. In 2004 an article in Nature magazine pointed out that "even small amounts of alcohol increase the risk of injury and boost the chances of developing about 60 diseases." In view of this, what constitutes safe drinking? Today millions of people worldwide safely enjoy having an occasional drink. The key to good health is moderation. But just what is moderation? Most people would consider their personal consumption to be moderate, perhaps reasoning that as long as they do not get drunk or are not alcohol dependent, there is no problem. Nevertheless, in Europe 1 man out of 4 has an alcohol consumption rate that is considered hazardous.

Various sources define moderate drinking as 0.70 ounce (20g) of pure alcohol per day, or two standard drinks for men, and 0.35 ounce (10g), or one drink, for women. French and British health authorities suggest "sensible limits" of three drinks per day for men and two for women. The U.S. National Institute on Alcohol Abuse and Alcoholism further recommends that "people aged 65 and older limit their consumption of alcohol to one drink per day." However, we all react differently to alcohol. In some cases, even these lower limits may be too high. For example, "moderate amounts of alcohol can be harmful to people with mood and anxiety disorders," notes the 10th Special Report to the U.S. Congress on Alcohol and Health. Age, medical history, and physique are factors to be taken into consideration.

Women who are breast-feeding should be aware that after they drink, alcohol builds up in their breast milk. In fact, the concentration of alcohol in breast milk is often higher than in blood, since there is more water in the milk to absorb the alcohol than there is in blood.

Since what is termed a "drink" varies from place to place, the amount of alcohol in a glass will reflect local standard servings and should be considered before consumption.

One for the Road
Restrictions on driving under the influence of alcohol have existed nearly as long as cars have. The first country to introduce such legislation was Denmark in 1903.

When you drink on an empty stomach, the alcohol in your blood reaches its highest level within about half an hour after it is ingested. Contrary to popular opinion, drinking coffee, taking in fresh air, and doing physical exercise will not help you to sober up. The only thing that will reduce the effect of alcohol on your body is the passing of time. Don't forget, too, that "a drink is a drink." That is, if you have a standard drink of wine, beer, or spirits, the alcohol content is the same.

Even small amounts of alcohol can impair your driving ability. Alcohol affects your eyesight. Road signs appear to be smaller. Peripheral vision as well as your ability to judge distances and to focus on distant objects is reduced. Information processing, reflexes, and coordination are slowed down.

If you have an accident after having imbibed alcohol, your injuries are likely to be more serious than if you had been sober. Moreover, your chances of surviving any emergency surgery diminish because of the effect of alcohol on the heart and the circulation. "Thus, contrary to generally accepted ideas, the majority of alcohol-related deaths are of drunk drivers themselves," notes a report by the French National Institute of Health and Medical Research. In view of the dangers, the report gives the following recommendations:

- Don't drink and drive.
- Don't get into a car with a driver who has been drinking.
- Don't let friends or parents drive under the influence of alcohol.

Generally speaking, about seven grams (0.25 ounce) of alcohol are eliminated per hour. A standard drink varies from country to country. *The World Health Organization defines a standard drink as containing 10 grams (0.35 ounce) of pure alcohol.* This is the approximate equivalent of 250 milliliters of beer (8 ounces), 100 milliliters of wine (3.4 ounces), or 30 milliliters (1 ounce) of spirits.

These drinks contain roughly the same amount of alcohol

A bottle of regular beer (330 ml [11 ounces] at 5% alcohol)
A single shot of spirits (whiskey, gin, vodka) (40 ml [1.4 ounces] at 40% alcohol)
A glass of wine (140 ml [5 ounces] at 12% alcohol)
A small glass of liqueur (70 ml [2.4 ounces] at 25% alcohol)

1.4.1. ALCOHOL DEPENDENCE — IS IT IN THE GENES
In a bid to find a treatment for alcoholism, scientists have striven to understand the role that genes play in its genesis and evolution. Scientists have since discovered several genes that seem to influence

one's reaction to alcohol. However, genetic factors are not the only ones in alcoholism. Even if some people do have a certain genetic predisposition, dependence is not inevitable. Environmental components are involved. Poor parenting, alcohol abuse in the home or by peers, situations involving conflict, emotional difficulties, depression, aggressiveness, thrill seeking, high resistance to alcohol's effects, or addiction to another substance have all been cited as risk factors. These and other elements open the way for dependence.

France:
Studies estimate that the number of people who abuse alcohol is some five million, of which between two and three million are alcohol dependent

Nigeria:
According to the Lagos newspaper Daily Champion, "over 15 million Nigerians are alcoholics"—that is nearly 12 percent of the population

Portugal:
This country has one of the world's highest per capita consumptions of pure alcohol. The Lisbon newspaper Público reports that 10 percent of the population suffers from "serious disabilities related to alcohol"

United States:
According to the 10th Special Report to the U.S. Congress on Alcohol and Health, "approximately 14 million Americans—7.4 percent of the population—meet the diagnostic criteria for alcohol abuse or alcoholism"

Limiting the Risk
The following definitions of low-risk limits were published by the Department of Mental Health and Substance Dependence of the World Health Organization. Low risk does not mean no risk. Individual reactions to alcohol vary.

- No more than two standard drinks a day
- On at least two days of the week, do not drink

In the following circumstances, even one or two drinks can be too much:

- When driving or operating machinery
- When pregnant or breast-feeding
- When taking certain medications
- When you have certain medical conditions
- If you cannot control your drinking

One standard drink equals 0.35 ounce (10g) of alcohol per unit or per glass.

Alcohol: Good for the Heart?

Scientists suspect that chemicals in red wine (polyphenols) inhibit a chemical that causes blood vessels to constrict.

Furthermore, alcohol in general has been linked to increased levels of so-called good cholesterol. It also reduces substances that can cause blood clots.

Any benefits from alcohol seem to involve drinking small amounts spread throughout the week, rather than the total amount all at once on a night out. Exceeding two drinks per day is linked to increases in blood pressure, and heavy drinking raises the risk of stroke and can cause swelling of the heart as well as irregular heartbeat. Immoderate drinking causes these and other health risks to outweigh any positive effects of alcohol on the cardiovascular system. Too much of a good thing is precisely that—too much.

1.4.2. HOW ALCOHOL CAN DAMAGE YOU

Brain

Cell loss, memory loss, depression, aggressive behavior

Vision, speech, coordination impairment

Cancer of throat, mouth, breast, liver

Heart
Muscle weakness, potential heart failure

Liver
Fatty, then enlarged, then scarred (cirrhosis)

Other risks
Poor immune system, ulcers, inflammation of pancreas.

Pregnant women
Risk of deformed or retarded babies: "Alcohol is far worse for the developing fetus than any other abused drug".

1.5. BREAKING THE CHAINS OF ALCOHOL ABUSE

Recognizing the Problem

First, it is imperative that the person who drinks alcohol and those close to him or her recognize it when a problem exists. Dependence is only the tip of the iceberg. It develops over a length of time from a pattern of drinking that was perhaps once moderate. Surprisingly, the majority of accidents, violence, and social difficulties caused by alcohol are not provoked by people who are compulsive alcohol drinkers. Note what the World Health Organization (WHO) says: *"The best way to reduce the total of alcohol-related problems in a society is to focus on curtailing the drinking of moderate rather than heavy drinkers."* Does your drinking exceed the limits recommended by health authorities? Do you drink in situations requiring your full attention and quick reflexes? Are your drinking habits causing problems in your family or at work? Acknowledging that one's level of consumption is potentially dangerous and reducing it accordingly is indeed "the best way" to avoid serious problems later. Once a person is dependent, it is far harder to make changes.

A common reaction among those who abuse alcohol is denial. "I drink like everyone else" or "I can stop whenever I want to," they claim.

How can a person be helped to recognize his drinking problem and then to take positive action? First, he has to admit that his difficulties arise from abuse of alcohol and that abstinence will improve his quality of life. As stated in *La Revue du Praticien—Médecine Générale,* his reasoning needs to change from "I drink because my wife left me and I lost my job," to "my wife left me and I lost my job because I drink."

If you want to help an alcohol-dependent person achieve this transformation in his thinking, you may want to follow these suggestions: Listen attentively, use open questions that allow the person to express his emotions and feelings freely, display an empathetic attitude that helps him feel that he is understood, give encouragement even for slight progress, avoid being judgmental or having an attitude that could block him from open expression and from seeking help. Having he or she write down two lists based on the questions: what will happen if I continue to drink? And what will happen if I stop? May also be useful.

Seeking Help

When someone begins to abuse alcohol, he or she is not worthless or beyond hope. Some even manage to break free on their own. However, individuals who are alcohol dependent may need professional help to become abstinent. For some people, outpatient treatment works, but when withdrawal symptoms are severe, hospitalization may be necessary. Once the initial physical withdrawal symptoms have passed—between two and five days—medication may be prescribed to reduce craving and to continue abstinence.

Detoxification programs, however, are no guarantee of success. Medication is only a temporary measure, not a cure. Dissociating with the same drinking partners and having the proper motivation to stop will enable someone to break the hold and hold out.

Filling the Void

In effect, many fail because the absence of alcohol leaves a void, somewhat like losing the companionship of a close friend. It is vital for the recovering alcoholic to find a new purpose in life if he is to stay abstinent.

A manual published by WHO with advice for those trying to change their drinking habits highlights the importance of purposeful activities in avoiding a relapse. One idea given as an example is engaging in religious activities.

Coping With a Relapse

Counselors on alcohol abuse point out the importance of support and encouragement for the recovering alcoholic. Many have lost family and friends because of their deplorable condition. The resulting isolation can lead to depression and even suicide. The manual mentioned above gives the following advice for those assisting someone with a drinking problem: "Try not to criticize the person you are helping, even if you get annoyed and frustrated with his or her behaviour. Remember that changing habits is never easy. There are bound to be good weeks and bad weeks. Your encouragement, support of low-risk drinking or abstinence, and creative ideas are needed."

If you are struggling to break free of alcohol, remember that relapses are likely to occur and that you should consider them as part of the road to recovery. Do not give up! Analyze what led to the relapse, and use that knowledge to prevent future slips. Identify specific situations that arouse in you the desire to drink. Could it be boredom, depression, loneliness, arguments, stress, or events or places where others drink? Then avoid them! "Learn to understand and identify the emotions that could lead to drinking and avoid any trigger situations. Stay away from places where people drink alcohol and even avoid body care products or medicines that are alcohol based.

Freedom

While it can be an ongoing challenge, escape from the shackles of alcohol dependence is possible. A person can make changes whether he is at risk of an accident through misuse of alcohol, is suffering problems because of abusing alcohol, or is alcohol dependent. If your drinking poses a threat to your well-being, do not hesitate to make the necessary changes. It can be for your own good and for the good of those who love you. There are many treatment centers, hospitals, and recovery programs that can provide help. Admitting the problem is the first step. Many need professional help to break free.

1.6. ALCOHOL MISUSE—A SOCIAL CATASTROPHE

The drinking of alcoholic beverages has two faces: one happy and the other sad. Let us take a closer look at the high cost of the misuse of alcohol.

Death Toll

Worldwide, the cost of alcohol misuse in terms of human life is incalculable. In France alcohol abuse is the third cause of death, after cancer and coronary heart disease, killing some 50,000 people directly or indirectly each year. This is "the equivalent of two to three jumbo-jet crashes each week," according to a report commissioned by the French Health Ministry.

The death toll exacted by alcohol is especially heavy among young people. According to a World Health Organization report published in 2001, alcohol is the leading cause of death among European men aged 15 to 29. It is predicted that soon in some Eastern European countries, misuse of alcohol will kill 1 out of every 3 young men there.

Violence and Sexual Assault

Alcohol contributes to acts of violence. Drinking can remove inhibitions and social restraints and can blur the way one interprets other people's actions, making a violent response more likely.

Alcohol is a significant factor in domestic violence and sexual assault. A French study of prison inmates suggested that alcohol was involved in two thirds of rapes and indecent assaults. Surveys indicate that in Poland, 75 percent of alcoholics' wives have been subjected to violence, notes the magazine *Polityka*. The authors of one study estimated that "the use of alcohol is associated with an approximately two-fold increased risk of homicide within all age groups and that (even) nondrinkers living in homes with alcohol users were at increased risk of homicide."—American Medical Association, Council on Scientific Affairs.

Social Cost

When health and insurance costs and lost productivity resulting from accidents, illness, or premature death are calculated, the financial cost to society is staggering. Alcohol abuse is said to cost Ireland's four million people at least one billion dollars a year. A source quoted in *The Irish Times* stated that this sum is equal to "the price of a new hospital, a sports stadium and a jet for every Minister every year." In 1998 the *Mainichi Daily News* reported that the economic impact of heavy drinking in Japan was "more than 6 trillion yen ($55 billion) a year." A report to the U.S. Congress declared: "The estimated economic cost of alcohol abuse was $184.6 billion for 1998 alone, or roughly $638 for every man, woman, and child living in the United States that year." And what about the psychological cost of broken or bereaved families and stunted educations or careers? The consequences to society of alcohol misuse are not hard to discern.

Do your drinking habits pose a risk to your health and to that of others?

CHAPTER 2

SUBSTANCE ABUSE, ADDICTION AND MISUSE

MANY PEOPLE DO not understand why or how other people become addicted to drugs. It is often mistakenly assumed that drug abusers lack moral principles or willpower and that they could stop using drugs simply by choosing to change their behavior. In reality, drug addiction is a complex disease, and quitting takes more than good intentions or a strong will. In fact, because drugs change the brain in ways that foster compulsive drug abuse, quitting is difficult, even for those who are ready to do so. Through scientific advances, we know more about how drugs work in the brain than ever, and we also know that drug addiction can be successfully treated to help people stop abusing drugs and lead productive lives.

2.1. DEFINITIONS OF SUBSTANCE ABUSE, ADDICTION AND MISUSE

Drug abuse, also called substance abuse or chemical abuse, is a disorder that is characterized by a destructive pattern of using a substance that leads to significant problems or distress.

Addiction is a physical and/or psychological need for a substance, due to regular, continued use. Some substances are highly addictive, others are less addictive. However, the symptoms of addiction are similar no matter which substance is used.

Substance misuse is the harmful use of substances (like drugs and alcohol) for non-medical purposes. The term "substance misuse" often refers to illegal drugs. However, legal substances can also be misused, such as alcohol, prescription medications, caffeine, nicotine and volatile substances (e.g. petrol, glue, paint).

Typical signs of substance misuse or addiction include:

- Neglecting responsibilities and activities you used to enjoy (e.g. work, family, hobbies, sports, socializing)
- Participating in dangerous or risky behaviours (e.g. drink driving, unprotected sex, using dirty needles)
- Criminal problems (e.g. disorderly behaviour, drink driving, stealing)
- Relationship problems (e.g. arguments with partner/family/friends, losing friends)
- Physical tolerance (e.g. needing more substance to experience the same effects, symptoms of withdrawal when not using)
- Losing control of your substance use (e.g. unable to stop using, even if you want to)
- Substance use takes over your life (e.g. spending a lot of time using, finding/getting drugs and recovering from the effects).

2.2. WHAT IS ABUSE AND MISUSE OF PRESCRIPTION DRUGS?

When a person takes a legal prescription medication for a purpose other than the reason it was prescribed, or when that person takes a drug not prescribed to him or her, that is misuse of a drug. Misuse can include taking a drug in a manner or at a dose that was not recommended by a health care professional. This can happen when the person hopes to get a bigger or faster therapeutic response from medications such as sleeping or weight loss pills. It can also happen when the person wants to "get high," which is an example of prescription drug abuse.

2.3. WHAT IS THE DIFFERENCE BETWEEN ABUSE AND MISUSE?

It mostly has to do with the individual's intentions or motivations. For example, let's say that a person knows that he will get a pleasant or euphoric feeling by taking the drug, especially at higher doses than prescribed. That is an example of drug abuse because the person is specifically looking for that euphoric response.

In contrast, if a person is not able to fall asleep after taking a single sleeping pill, they may take another pill an hour later, thinking, "That will do the job." Or a person may offer his headache medication to a friend who is in pain. Those are examples of drug misuse because, even though these people did not follow medical instructions, they were not looking to "get high" from the drugs. They were treating themselves, but not according to the directions of their health care providers.

However, no matter the intention of the person, both misuse and abuse of prescription drugs can be harmful and even life-threatening to the individual. This is because taking a drug other than the way it is prescribed can lead to dangerous outcomes that the person may not anticipate.

2.4. WHY DO PEOPLE MISUSE SUBSTANCE?

People use drugs and alcohol for many reasons. We might use substances to relax, have fun, cope with or escape a problem or dull emotional/physical pain. However, using substances to cope with problems or numb your pain does not make the problems go away and can make them worse. Also, you might come to depend on drugs or alcohol as a way of coping, rather than seeking help and finding more positive strategies and solutions.

2.5. WHAT HAPPENS TO YOUR BRAIN WHEN YOU TAKE DRUGS?

Drugs contain chemicals that tap into the brain's communication system and disrupt the way nerve cells normally send, receive, and process information. There are at least two ways that drugs cause this disruption: (1) by imitating the brain's natural chemical messengers and (2) by over-stimulating the "reward circuit" of the brain.

Some drugs (e.g., marijuana and heroin) have a similar structure to chemical messengers called neurotransmitters, which are naturally produced by the brain. This similarity allows the drugs to "fool" the brain's receptors and activate nerve cells to send abnormal messages.

Other drugs, such as cocaine or methamphetamine, can cause the nerve cells to release abnormally large amounts of natural neurotransmitters (mainly dopamine) or to prevent the normal recycling of these brain chemicals, which is needed to shut off the signaling between neurons. The result is a brain awash in dopamine, a neurotransmitter present in brain regions that control movement, emotion, motivation, and feelings of pleasure. The overstimulation of this reward system, which normally responds to natural behaviors linked to survival (eating, spending time with loved ones, etc.), produces euphoric effects in response to psychoactive drugs. This reaction sets in motion a reinforcing pattern that "teaches" people to repeat the rewarding behavior of abusing drugs.

As a person continues to abuse drugs, the brain adapts to the overwhelming surges in dopamine by producing less dopamine or by reducing the number of dopamine receptors in the reward circuit. The result is a lessening of dopamine's impact on the reward circuit, which reduces the abuser's ability to enjoy not only the drugs but also other events in life that previously brought pleasure. This decrease compels the addicted person to keep abusing drugs in an attempt to bring the dopamine function back to normal, but now larger amounts of the drug are required to achieve the same dopamine high—an effect known as tolerance.

Long-term abuse causes changes in other brain chemical systems and circuits as well. Glutamate is a neurotransmitter that influences the reward circuit and the ability to learn. When the optimal concentration of glutamate is altered by drug abuse, the brain attempts to compensate, which can impair cognitive function. Brain imaging studies of drug-addicted individuals show changes in areas of the brain that are critical to judgment, decision making, learning and memory, and behavior control. Together, these changes can drive an abuser to seek out and take drugs compulsively despite adverse, even devastating consequences—that is the nature of addiction.

2.6 WHY DO SOME PEOPLE BECOME ADDICTED WHILE OTHERS DO NOT?

No single factor can predict whether a person will become addicted to drugs. Risk for addiction is influenced by a combination of factors that include individual biology, social environment, and age or stage of development. The more risk factors an individual has, the greater the chance that taking drugs can lead to addiction. For example:

Biology: The genes that people are born with in combination with environmental influences account for about half of their addiction vulnerability. Additionally, gender, ethnicity, and the presence of other mental disorders may influence risk for drug abuse and addiction.

Environment: A person's environment includes many different influences, from family and friends to socioeconomic status and quality of life in general. Factors such as peer pressure, physical and sexual abuse, stress, and quality of parenting can greatly influence the occurrence of drug abuse and the escalation to addiction in a person's life.

Development: Genetic and environmental factors interact with critical developmental stages in a person's life to affect addiction vulnerability. Although taking drugs at any age can lead to addiction, the earlier that drug use begins, the more likely it will progress to more serious abuse, which poses a special challenge to adolescents. Because areas in their brains that govern decision making, judgment, and self-control are still developing, adolescents may be especially prone to risk-taking behaviors, including trying drugs of abuse.

2.7. SOME DRUGS FEATURES, HEALTH EFFECTS AND TREATMENT OPTIONS

Cannabis (Marijuana)

Greenish-gray mixture of the dried, shredded leaves, stems, seeds, and/or flowers of Cannabis sativa or cannabis indica—the hemp plant

Health Effects

Acute	Heightened sensory perception; euphoria, followed by drowsiness/relaxation; impaired short-term memory, attention, judgment, coordination and balance; increased heart rate; increased appetite
Long-term	Addiction: About 9 percent of users; about 1 in 6 of those who started using in their teens; 25 to 50 % of daily users. Mental disorders: may be a causal factor in schizophreniform disorders (in those with a pre-existing vulnerability); is associated with depression and anxiety.
	Smoking related: chronic cough; bronchitis; lung and upper airway cancers is undetermined.
In combination with alcohol	Magnified tachychardia and effect on blood pressure; amplified impairment of cognitive, psychomotor, and driving performance
Withdrawal symptoms	Irritability, difficulty sleeping, strange nightmares, craving, and anxiety.

Associated Special Vulnerabilities/Populations

Youth	Almost 44 percent of teens have tried marijuana by the time they graduate from high school (MTF, 2010)

Treatment options

Medications	There are no FDA-approved medications to treat marijuana addiction.
Behavioral Therapies	• Cognitive-behavioral therapy (CBT) • Contingency management, or motivational incentives • Motivational Enhancement Therapy (MET) • Behavioral treatments geared to adolescents (For more information on these treatments, please see NIDA's Principles of Drug Addiction Treatment: A Research-Based Guide - Behavioral Therapies.)

Cocaine

White crystalline powder that can be snorted, injected or smoked

Health Effects

Acute	Dilated pupils; increased body temperature, heart rate, and blood pressure; nausea; increased energy, alertness; euphoria; decreased appetite and sleep.
	High doses: Erratic and violent behavior, panic attacks
Long-term	Addiction, restlessness, anxiety, irritability, paranoia, panic attacks, mood disturbances; insomnia; nasal damage and difficulty swallowing from snorting; GI problems; HIV
In combination with alcohol	When combined, there is a greater risk of overdose and sudden death than either drug alone.
Withdrawal symptoms	Depression, fatigue, increased appetite, insomnia or hypersomnia, vivid unpleasant dreams, psychomotor retardation or agitation

Associated Special Vulnerabilities/Populations

Pregnancy	Premature delivery, low birth weights, and smaller for gestational age.

Treatment options

Medications	There are no FDA-approved medications to treat cocaine addiction.
Behavioral Therapies	• Cognitive-behavioral therapy (CBT) • Community reinforcement approach plus vouchers • Contingency management, or motivational incentives The matrix model • 12-Step facilitation therapy (For more information on these treatments, please see NIDA's Principles of Drug Addiction Treatment: A Research-Based Guide - Behavioral Therapies.)

Prescription Stimulants (Abuse)

Amphetamine (Dexedrine, Adderall), Methylphenidate (Ritalin, Concerta)

Health Effects

Acute	Increased alertness, attention, energy; irregular heartbeat, dangerously high body temperature, potential for cardiovascular failure or seizures.
Long-term	High doses especially, or alternate routes of administration (e.g., snorting, injecting) can lead to anxiety, hostility, paranoia, psychosis; addiction.

In combination with alcohol	Masks the depressant action of alcohol, increasing risk of alcohol overdose. May increase blood pressure; jitters.
Withdrawal symptoms	Depression, fatigue, increased appetite, insomnia or hypersomnia, vivid unpleasant dreams, psychomotor retardation or agitation

Associated Special Vulnerabilities/Populations

Female adolescents	Unlike some illicit drugs and alcohol, stimulants are used at equal or greater frequency by young females vs. males. Use is often to lose weight, stay awake to study, or perform better on exams.
Mixing with antidepressants or OTC cold medicines	May enhance adverse effects; cause blood pressure to become dangerously high or lead to irregular heart rhythms.

Treatment options

Medications	There are no FDA-approved medications to treat stimulant addiction.
Behavioral Therapies	Behavioral therapies that have proven effective for treating addiction to illicit stimulant drugs, such as cocaine and methamphetamine, may be useful in addressing prescription stimulant addiction. (For more information on these treatments, please see NIDA's Principles of Drug Addiction Treatment: A Research-Based Guide - Behavioral Therapies.)

Methamphetamine

White, odorless, bitter-tasting crystalline powder that is easily dissolved in water or alcohol; can be ingested orally, intranasally, injected, or smoked

Health Effects

Acute	Enhanced mood; increased heart rate, blood pressure, body temperature, energy and activity; decreased appetite; dry mouth; increased sexuality; jaw-clenching
Long-term	Addiction, memory loss; weight loss; impaired cognition; insomnia, anxiety, irritability, confusion, paranoia, aggression, mood disturbances, hallucinations, violent behavior; liver, kidney, lung damage; severe dental problems; cardiac and neurological damage; HIV, Hepatitis

Withdrawal symptoms	Depression, anxiety, fatigue, and intense craving for the drug.

Associated Special Vulnerabilities/Populations

Pregnancy	Increased risk of premature birth, placental abruption, fetal growth retardation, and heart and brain abnormalities

Treatment options

Medications	There are no FDA-approved medications to treat methamphetamine addiction.
Behavioral Therapies	• Cognitive-behavioral therapy (CBT) • Contingency management, or motivational incentives • The matrix model • 12-Step facilitation therapy (For more information on these treatments, please see NIDA's Principles of Drug Addiction Treatment: A Research-Based Guide - Behavioral Therapies.)

Inhalants

Volatile solvents, Aerosols, Gases, Nitrites (Poppers). Effects depend on the properties of the chemical, but inhalation is the common route of abuse

Health Effects

Acute	Confusion; nausea; slurred speech; lack of coordination; euphoria; dizziness; drowsiness; disinhibition, lightheadedness, hallucinations/delusions;headaches; suffocation; convulsions/seizures; hypoxia; heart failure; coma; sudden sniffing death (butane, propane, and other chemicals in aerosols) **Nitrites** - Systemic vasodilation; increased heart rate; brief sensation of heat and excitement; dizziness; headache.
Long-term	Myelin break down leading to muscle spasms, tremors and possible permanent motor impairment; liver/kidney damage. Addiction - A minority inhale on a regular basis, but among those, some report symptoms of addiction (need to continue using, despite severe adverse consequences).

	Nitrites - HIV/AIDS and hepatitis; lipoid pneumonia
In combination with alcohol	**Nitrites** – Increased risk of adverse cardiovascular effects. Alcohol may increase the blood-vessel relaxant effect of organic nitrates (such as amyl nitrite) and result in dangerously low blood pressure.
Withdrawal symptoms	A mild withdrawal syndrome (e.g., irritability, restlessness, insomnia, headaches, poor concentration) can occur with long-term inhalant abuse.

Associated Special Vulnerabilities/Populations

Youth	Abused mostly by younger (8th graders) rather than older teens (10th and 12th graders)
	Nitrites have been linked to high risk sexual behaviors and HIV transmission. Because of their vasodilating actions on the anal sphincter, they are frequently used to facilitate anal intercourse by men who have sex with men.
Pregnancy	Although rigorous studies have not been conducted, data from occupational exposure to abused solvents like toluene suggest increased spontaneous abortion and fetal malformations.

Treatment options

Medications	There are no FDA-approved medications to treat inhalant addiction
Behavioral Therapies	There are no published reports of behavioral approaches for the treatment of inhalant abuse.

Prescription Sedatives, sleeping pills*, or anxiolytics (Abuse)

Central nervous system depressants include barbiturates (e.g., Nembutal) and benzodiazepines (e.g., Valium, Xanax)

Health Effects

Acute	Drowsiness, relaxation, overdose
Long-term	Tolerance, physical dependence, addiction
In combination with alcohol	Slows both heart rate and respiration, which can be fatal
Withdrawal symptoms	Discontinuing prolonged use, absent a physician's guidance can lead to serious withdrawal symptoms, including seizures. For barbiturates, abrupt cessation can be life-threatening.

Treatment options

Medications	Addicted patients should undergo medically supervised detoxification because the treatment dose must be gradually tapered.
Behavioral Therapies	Behavioral therapies, such as cognitive behavioral therapy, that have proven effective for treating addiction to other illicit substances may be useful in addressing addiction to prescription sedatives.
	(For more information on these treatments, please see NIDA's Principles of Drug Addiction Treatment: A Research-Based Guide - Behavioral Therapies.)

2.8. SOLUTIONS TO DRUG PROBLEMS

Recognize when your substance use becomes a problem – realizing and accepting that you are misusing or addicted to a substance is the first step in finding solutions.

Get support – getting through substance misuse and addiction on your own is very difficult. Talking to family members, friends, your doctor, other health professionals or a telephone helpline (such as Lifeline) about your substance or drug use can help you to feel supported, find appropriate treatment options and assist in your recovery.

Investigate treatment options – there are many ways to manage substance or drug misuse and addiction, including some free and low cost options. Types of support include counseling, medication, rehabilitation centers, self-help programs, support networks and others. Talk to a helpline or doctor about available services. Everyone responds differently, so you may need to try a number of options to find what works for you.

Find alternative coping strategies – often people use substances to cope with or escape other personal problems. Finding positive ways of managing stress and problems will help you to manage your substance use and prevent relapses.

Dealing with setbacks – recovery from substance addiction is a long road and sometimes you may experience setbacks. Rather than giving up or feeling like a failure following a relapse, try to get back on the wagon as quickly as possible. It also helps to figure out what triggered the relapse and how you can change your behavior in the future.

The reader is advised to carefully consult the instruction and information material included in the package insert of each drug or therapeutic agent before administration.
This advice is especially important when using, administering, or recommending new and infrequently used drugs.

CHAPTER 3

DIET, DIABETES AND NUTRITION

3.1. DIET

IN NUTRITION, DIET is the sum of food consumed by a person or other organism. Dietary habits are the habitual decisions an individual or culture makes when choosing what foods to eat. The word diet often implies the use of specific intake of nutrition for health or weight-management reasons (with the two often being related). Although humans are omnivores, each culture and each person holds some food preferences or some food taboos. This may be due to personal tastes or ethical reasons. Individual dietary choices may be more or less healthy.

Proper nutrition requires ingestion and absorption of vitamins, minerals, and food energy in the form of carbohydrates, proteins, and fats. Dietary habits and choices play a significant role in the quality of life, health and longevity. It can define cultures and play a role in religion.

Religious and cultural dietary choices
Some cultures and religions have restrictions concerning what foods are acceptable in their diet. For example, only Kosher foods are permitted by Judaism, and Halal foods by Islam. Although Buddhists are generally vegetarians, the practice varies and meat-eating may be permitted depending on the sects. In Hinduism, vegetarianism is the ideal, Jain is strictly vegetarian and consumption of roots is not permitted.

Dietary choices
Many people choose to forgo food from animal sources to varying degrees (e.g. flexitarianism, vegetarianism, veganism, fruitarianism) for health reasons, issues surrounding morality, or to reduce their personal impact on the environment, although some of the public assumptions about which diets have lower impacts are known to be incorrect. Raw foodism is another contemporary trend. These diets may require tuning or supplementation such as vitamins to meet ordinary nutritional needs.

Weight management
A particular diet may be chosen to seek weight loss or weight gain. Changing a subject's dietary intake, or "going on a diet", can change the energy balance and increase or decrease the amount of fat stored by the body. Some foods are specifically recommended, or even altered, for conformity to the requirements of a particular diet. These diets are often recommended in conjunction with exercise. Specific weight loss programs can be harmful to health, while others may be beneficial (and can thus be coined as healthy diets). *The terms "healthy diet" and "diet for weight management" are often related, as the two promote healthy weight management.* Having a healthy diet is a way to prevent health problems, and will provide your body with the right balance of vitamins, minerals, and other nutrients.

Eating disorders
An eating disorder is a mental disorder that interferes with normal food consumption. It is defined by abnormal eating habits that may involve either insufficient or excessive diet.

Healthy diet
A healthy diet may improve or maintain optimal health. In developed countries, affluence enables unconstrained caloric intake and possibly inappropriate food choices.

It is recommended by many authorities that people maintain a normal weight by (limiting consumption of energy-dense foods and sugary drinks), eat plant-based food, limit red and processed meat, and limit alcohol. However, there is no total consensus on what constitutes a healthy diet.

Table 3.1: Diet classification

	Carnivorous	Ketogenic	Omnivorous	Pescetarian	Vegetarian	Vegan	Raw vegan	Islamic	Hindu	Jewish	Paleolithic	Fruitarian
Fruits and berries	No	No	Yes	Yes	Yes	Yes	Yes	Yes	Yes	Yes	Yes	Yes
Greens	No	Maybe	Yes	Yes	Yes	Yes	Yes	Yes	Yes	Yes	Yes	Yes
Vegetables	No	No	Yes	Yes	Yes	Yes	Yes	Yes	Yes	Yes	Yes	No
Legumes	No	No	Yes	Yes	Yes	Yes	Yes	Yes	Yes	Yes	No	No
Tubers	No	No	Yes	Yes	Yes	Yes	No	Yes	Yes	Yes	Yes	No
Grains	No	No	Yes	Yes	Yes	Yes	No	Yes	Yes	Yes	No	No
Poultry	Yes	Yes	Yes	No	No	No	No	Yes	No	Yes	Yes	No
Fish (scaled)	Yes	Yes	Yes	Yes	No	No	No	Yes	No	Yes	Yes	No
Seafood (non-fish)	Yes	Yes	Yes	Yes	No	No	No	Yes	No	No	Yes	No
Beef	Yes	Yes	Yes	No	No	No	No	Yes	No	Yes	Yes	No
Pork	Yes	Yes	Yes	No	No	No	No	No	No	No	Yes	No
Eggs	Yes	Yes	Yes	Yes	Maybe	No	No	Yes	No	Yes	Yes	No
Dairy	No	Maybe	Yes	Yes	Maybe	No	No	Yes	Yes	Yes	No	No
Nuts	No	Maybe	Yes	Yes	Yes	Yes	Yes	Yes	Yes	Yes	Yes	Yes
Alcohol	No	Maybe	Yes	Yes	Yes	Yes	No	No	No	Yes	No	No

3.2. CLASSIFICATION OF FOOD

On the basis of nutrients, food can be classified into seven different groups:

- Carbohydrates
- Proteins
- Fats
- Vitamins
- Minerals
- Fibre or Roughage
- Water

Table 3.2: Composition of some common foods

Food	Carbohydrate	Fat	Protein
Bread(Chapatti)	52%	3%	9%
Rice(cooked)	23%	0.1%	2.2%
Banana	20%	0.5%	1.0%
Apple	12.8%	0.5%	0.3%
Egg	0.7%	12%	13%
Milk	4%	4%	3%
Butter	0.4%	81%	0.6%
Meat	0	30%	22%

3.2.1. CARBOHYDRATES

Carbohydrates are compounds of carbon, hydrogen and oxygen. According to their chemical structure they may be simple or complex. Sugar and starch are complex where as glucose is simple.

Carbohydrates are the body's main source of energy. There are two types of carbohydrates: simple and complex.

- **Simple carbohydrates** are found in fruits, vegetables, and milk products, as well as in sweeteners like sugar, honey, and syrup and foods like candy, soft drinks, and frosting or icing.
- **Complex carbohydrates** are found in breads, cereals, pasta, rice, beans and peas, and starchy vegetables such as potatoes, green peas, and corn.

Many carbohydrates also supply fiber. Fiber is a type of complex carbohydrate found in foods that come from plants—fruits, vegetables, nuts, seeds, beans, and whole grains. Eating food with fiber can prevent stomach or intestinal problems, such as constipation. It might also help lower cholesterol and blood sugar.

In the process of digestion, cooked starch, by the action of enzymes, breaks down into glucose. Glucose is very easily assimilated by the intestine and sent to every part of the body. On reaching the cells, glucose gets oxidized to release energy. ***One gram of carbohydrate yields 4.2 calories of energy.*** Hence the function of carbohydrates is to supply energy to the body for work and other physiological activities.

Example: Rice, wheat, maize, bajra, ragi, potato, sweet potato, tapioca, banana, sugarcane etc.

3.2.2. Proteins

Proteins are often called the body's building blocks. They are used to build and repair tissues. They are complex compounds made up of chains of nitrogen containing building blocks called amino acids. Besides nitrogen they also contain carbon, hydrogen and oxygen. They help you fight infection. Your body uses extra protein for energy. The proteins present in living organisms contain more than 20 amino acids and each of them has a specific function.

Table 4: Functions of some proteins

Type of body proteins	Functions
Enzymes	Biocatalysts, i.e. help in biochemical reactions occurring in the body all the time Example : pepsin
Transport Proteins	carry different substances in the blood to different tissues Example : Haemoglobin
Contractile proteins	Responsible for muscle contraction for movement and locomotion Example : Myosin
Hormones	Some hormones are proteins. Hormones regulate body functions Example : Insulin
Structural Proteins	form parts of cells and tissues Example : Collagen
Protective proteins	Help fight Infections. Example Antibodies, Gamma globulins

Proteins, being highly complex compounds, cannot be used by our body in this form. By the action of digestive enzymes, proteins are broken down into simpler form i.e. amino acids which are assimilated into the blood in the intestine. The blood carries these free amino acids to the various body cells where they are regrouped to form specific proteins such as skin, muscles, blood and bones. Thus proteins are essential for body growth and functioning. Deficiency of protein causes retardation of physical and mental growth. The two PEM (Protein Energy Malnutrition) diseases are Kwashiorkor and Marasmus found in children. Good sources of protein are seafood, lean meat and poultry, eggs, beans and peas, soy products, cheese, pulses (dal) and unsalted nuts and seeds. Protein is also found in dairy products. Protein from plant sources tends to be lower in fat and cholesterol and provides fiber and other health-promoting nutrients.

3.2.3. FATS

Fats are substances that are not soluble in water. They are composed of fatty acids and glycerol. Fats are also called lipids. Fats also give you energy and help you feel satisfied after eating. Oils, shortening, butter, and margarine are types of fats, and mayonnaise, salad dressings, table cream, and sour cream are high in fat. Foods from animal sources and certain foods like seeds, nuts, avocado, and coconut also contain fat.

Sources of fat include animal meat, fish, and vegetable oils. Fats are used by the body:

- In every cell structure.
- Especially to build nerves and brain. The brain is 40% fat.
- To insulate the body.
- To produce sex hormones and adrenal cortex hormone
- To produce cholesterol (essential for cell membranes and bile salts, for example).
- To absorb certain vitamins (A, D, E, and K).
- To store energy.

There are different categories of fats—some are healthier than others:

- **Monounsaturated.** These include canola oil, olive oil, peanut oil, and safflower oil. They are found in avocados, peanut butter, and some nuts and seeds.
- **Polyunsaturated.** Some are corn oil, soybean oil, and flaxseed oil. They are also found in fatty fish, walnuts, and some seeds.
- **Saturated.** These fats are found in red meat, milk products including butter, and palm and coconut oils. Regular cheese, pizza, and grain-based and dairy desserts are common sources of saturated fat in our meals.
- **Trans fats (trans fatty acids).** Processed trans fats are found in stick margarine and vegetable shortening. Trans fats are often used in store-bought baked goods and fried foods at some fast-food restaurants.

You can identify monounsaturated and polyunsaturated fats because they are liquid at room temperature. These types of fat seem to lower your chance of heart disease. But that does not mean you can eat more than the Dietary Guidelines suggest.

Trans fats and saturated fats are usually solid at room temperature. Trans fat and saturated fat can put you at greater risk for heart disease and should be limited.

Cholesterol

Cholesterol is a fat-like substance found in some foods. Your body needs some cholesterol. But research suggests that eating a lot of foods high in saturated fat is associated with higher levels of cholesterol in your blood, which may increase your risk of heart disease. Try to limit cholesterol to less than 300 mg each day. If your doctor says you need to lower your cholesterol, you might need to limit cholesterol in your food to less than 200 mg each day.

Carbohydrates, proteins, and fats supply 90% of the dry weight of the diet and 100% of its energy. All three provide energy (measured in calories), but the amount of energy in 1 gram (1/28 ounce) differs:

- *4 calories in a gram of carbohydrate or protein*
- *9 calories in a gram of fat*

These nutrients also differ in how quickly they supply energy. Carbohydrates are the quickest, and fats are the slowest.

Carbohydrates, proteins, and fats are digested in the intestine, where they are broken down into their basic units:

- *Carbohydrates into sugars*
- *Proteins into amino acids*
- *Fats into fatty acids and glycerol*

The body uses these basic units to build substances it needs for growth, maintenance, and activity (including other carbohydrates, proteins, and fats).

3.2.4. VITAMINS

Vitamins are substances that are required in the diet for health and wellbeing. Your body needs small amounts of vitamins for growth, reproduction and to maintain overall good health. There are a total of 13 vitamins that are divided into two categories based on how your body absorbs them. Water-soluble vitamins, which include vitamin C and the B vitamins niacin, thiamine, riboflavin, vitamin B-6, vitamin B-12, folate, biotin and pantothenic acid, are absorbed with water and enter your bloodstream directly. The fat-soluble vitamins, which include vitamin A, vitamin D, vitamin E and vitamin K, need dietary fat to be absorbed properly. The fat-soluble vitamins pass through your small intestine and into your lymphatic system before ultimately entering your bloodstream.

Vitamin deficiencies may result in disease conditions: goiter, scurvy, osteoporosis, impaired immune system, disorders of cell metabolism, certain forms of cancer, symptoms of premature aging, and poor psychological health (including eating disorders), among many others. Excess of some vitamins is also dangerous to health (notably vitamin A), and for at least one vitamin, B6, toxicity begins at levels not far above the required amount.

Storage of Vitamins
Your body has the ability to store fat-soluble vitamins. Vitamin A, K and E are stored in your liver and vitamin D is stored in your fat and muscle tissues. Your body releases some of the stored vitamins to meet your needs when your dietary intake of these vitamins falls short. Your body does not have the ability to store water-soluble vitamins. When you eat these vitamins, any excess is excreted in your urine. Because of this, fat-soluble vitamin deficiencies are less common than water-soluble vitamin deficiencies.

Vitamins and minerals occur in a variety of foods. That is, by eating a variety of foods, you can get the necessary vitamins and minerals you need for health.

3.2.5. MINERALS

Minerals are non-organic or inorganic substances that are required in the diet. While only small amounts of minerals are required in our diet, they are critical in building bones and teeth, regulating heartbeat and transporting oxygen from the lungs to the tissues.

Minerals are divided into two classes – major and trace – based on how much your body needs to function properly. You need the major minerals in larger amounts, usually from hundreds to thousands of milligrams daily, while you only need the trace minerals in small amounts, usually less than 20 milligrams daily. The major minerals include sodium, potassium, chloride, calcium, phosphorus, magnesium and sulfur. The trace minerals include iron, zinc, iodine, selenium, fluoride, chromium, manganese, molybdenum and copper.

Essential dietary minerals

- Chlorine as chloride ions; very common electrolyte; see sodium, below

37

- Magnesium, required for processing ATP and related reactions (builds bone, causes strong peristalsis, increases flexibility, increases alkalinity). Approximately 50% is in bone, the remaining 50% is almost all inside body cells, and with only about 1% located in extracellular fluid. Food sources include oats, buckwheat, tofu, nuts, caviar, green leafy vegetables, legumes, and chocolate.
- Phosphorus, required component of bones; essential for energy processing. Approximately 80% is found in inorganic portion of bones and teeth. Phosphorus is a component of every cell, as well as important metabolites, including DNA, RNA, ATP, and phospholipids. Also important in pH regulation. Food sources include cheese, egg yolk, milk, meat, fish, poultry, whole-grain cereals, and many others.
- Potassium, a very common electrolyte (heart and nerve health). With sodium, potassium is involved in maintaining normal water balance, osmotic equilibrium, and acid-base balance. In addition to calcium, it is important in the regulation of neuromuscular activity. Food sources include bananas, avocados, vegetables, potatoes, legumes, and mushrooms.
- Sodium, a very common electrolyte; not generally found in dietary supplements, despite being needed in large quantities, because the ion is very common in food: typically as sodium chloride, or common salt

Trace minerals
Many elements are required in smaller amounts (microgram quantities), usually because they play a catalytic role in enzymes. Some trace mineral elements (RDA < 200 mg/day) are, in alphabetical order:

- Cobalt required for biosynthesis of vitamin B12 family of coenzymes.
- Copper required component of many redox enzymes, including cytochrome oxidase.

- Chromium required for sugar metabolism.
- Iodine required not only for the biosynthesis of thyroxin, but probably, for other important organs as breast, stomach, salivary glands, thymus etc. For this reason iodine is needed in larger quantities than others in this list, and sometimes classified with the macrominerals.
- Iron required for many enzymes, and for hemoglobin and some other proteins.
- Manganese (processing of oxygen).
- Molybdenum required for xanthine oxidase and related oxidases.
- Nickel present in urease.
- Selenium required for peroxidase (antioxidant proteins).
- Zinc required for several enzymes such as carboxypeptidase, liver alcohol dehydrogenase and carbonic anhydrase.

Deficiency or excess of minerals can also have serious health consequences.

3.2.6. FIBER OR ROUGHAGE

Fiber or roughage: refers to the non-digestible carbohydrates in vegetables and to a lesser extent in fruit. Fibre may actually be 'fibrous', as in celery, or may be a powder, or, when mixed with water in the intestines, a jelly. Fibre provides:

- Bulk
- Lubrication, and
- Nutrition for friendly bacteria in the colon.

When fibre is combined with water, it swells up and provides bulk to the digestive system. This makes it easier for food to pass through the intestines. Food also passes through the digestive system faster, so that waste products are retained for less time in the body.

Some fibre has the effect of lubricating the contents of the intestines and, therefore, makes the food pass through easily and in a timely manner. The benefits here are the same as for bulk.

In addition, friendly bacteria in the colon feed on fibre and they are therefore nourished by it. By helping these friendly bacteria, we enable them to help us to digest food. Also, by giving them support, they are more able to exclude other, less friendly bacteria, from our colons. Fibre is, therefore, necessary for a healthy and efficient digestive system.

Dietary fiber is a carbohydrate (or a polysaccharide) that is incompletely absorbed in humans and in some animals. Like all carbohydrates, when it is metabolized it can produce four calories (kilocalories) of energy per gram. But in most circumstances it accounts for less than that because of its limited absorption and digestibility. There are two subcategories: insoluble and soluble fiber. Insoluble dietary fiber consists mainly of cellulose, a large carbohydrate polymer that is indigestible by humans who do not have the required enzymes to disassemble it nor do their digestive systems harbor sufficient quantities of the types of microbes that can do so either. Soluble dietary fiber comprises a variety of oligosaccharides, waxes, esters, resistant starches and other carbohydrates that dissolve or gelatinize in water. Many of these soluble fibers can be fermented or partially fermented by microbes in the human digestive system to produce short-chain fatty acids which are absorbed and therefore introduce some caloric content.

Whole grains, beans and other legumes, fruits (especially plums, prunes, and figs), and vegetables are good sources of dietary fiber. Fiber is important to digestive health and is thought to reduce the risk of colon cancer. For mechanical reasons it can help in alleviating both constipation and diarrhea. Fiber provides bulk to the intestinal contents, and insoluble fiber especially stimulates peristalsis – the rhythmic muscular contractions of the intestines which move digesta along the digestive tract. Some soluble fibers produce a solution of high viscosity; this is essentially a gel, which slows the movement of food through the intestines. Additionally, fiber, perhaps especially that from whole grains, may help lessen insulin spikes and reduce the risk of type 2 diabetes.

3.2.7. WATER

Water is one of the most important nutrients in the sports diet. It helps eliminate food waste products in the body, regulates body temperature during activity and helps with digestion. Maintaining hydration during periods of physical exertion is the key to peak performance. While drinking too much water during activities can lead to physical discomfort, dehydration in excess of 2% of body mass (by weight) markedly hinders athletic performance. Water and salt dosage is based on work performed, lean body mass, and environmental factors, especially ambient temperature and humidity. Maintaining the right amount is the key.

Health benefits of warm water
Six ways drinking warm water can heal your body
Regularly drinking very warm water instead of hot cup of coffee or tea to warm our bodies after getting out of bed or especially in the morning can heal our bodies, providing digestive power and reducing metabolic waste that could have built up in our immune system.

"Physicians recommend drinking warm water in the morning, usually, with a polyphenol-rich lemon immersion, or with a tea shown to decrease free radical activity in the body." -Medical Daily

The consumption of warm water increases the tightening of the intestines, which optimizes elimination. Unlike hot water, processed cold water is devoid of many essential minerals that could become very unfavorable to the digestive tract when consuming a meal.

While drinking warm water may not suit your taste buds, it may be beneficial to put the caffeine and tea aside for your health's sake. Here are six reasons why:

1. Cleanses Digestion
    A very warm cup of water in the morning can help cleanse your body by flushing out toxins. Water and other liquids help break down the food in your stomach and keep the digestive system on

track. Warm water will help break down these foods even faster, making them easier for you to digest. Drinking cold water during or after a meal can actually harden the oil in consumed foods and therefore create a fat deposit in the intestine. Adding ice to processed cold water will strip it of natural-containing minerals as these minerals are essential to keeping the digestive tract healthy. Replace a glass of cold water with a warm one to aid digestion, especially after eating a meal.

2. Aids Constipation

   At one point or another, many of us are plagued by this common stomach problem where we have little to no bowel movement. The strain felt during elimination, accompanied by bloating, is brought on by a lack of water in the body. Drinking very warm water in the morning on an empty stomach can help improve bowel movements and aid constipation while breaking down foods as they smoothly pass through the intestines. Stimulating the bowels will help return your body back to normal functioning.

3. Alleviates Pain

   Warm water, considered to be nature's most powerful home remedy, can help alleviate pain from menstruation to headaches. The heat from warm water is known to have a calming and soothing effect on the abdominal muscles, which can help provide instant relief for cramps and muscle spasms. According to Healthline, warm or hot water is usually better for cramps, as hot liquids increase blood flow to the skin and help relax the cramped muscles.

4. Sheds Excess Pounds

   Drinking a glass of warm water first thing in the morning can help with weight loss. Warm water increases body temperature, which therefore increases the metabolic rate. An increase in metabolic rate allows the body to burn more calories throughout the rate. It can also help the gastrointestinal tract and kidneys to function even better. Drinking a glass of warm water and a lemon will help break down the adipose tissue, or body fat, in your body, and also control food craving due to lemon's pectin fiber.

5. Improves Blood Circulation

The fat deposits in the body are eliminated along with accumulating deposits in the nervous system when you drink a glass of warm water. This flushes out the toxins that are circulating throughout the body and then enhances blood circulation. Making sure the muscles are relaxed, eliminate poor circulation and blood flow.

6. Halts Premature Aging

Premature aging is a woman's worst nightmare, but luckily, this can be prevented by drinking warm water. The presence of toxins in the body can lead to aging faster, but warm water can help cleanse the body from those toxins, while repairing skin cells to increase elasticity.

To reap the health benefits of warm water, drink it every morning plain or with a lemon for taste. Drinking straight hot water can potentially be damaging to tissue in the mouth and esophagus. After boiling water, be sure to let it cool for a few minutes before you start consuming. Also, "always check with your prescribing physician before drinking warm water if you're on any medications that could impact the efficacy of your medications.

Do not drink cold water

Most people like to drink cold water especially during summers. Their normal meals usually end up with a glass of cold water, a bottle of Pepsi-Cola or Coca-Cola etc. This is mostly for the taste and enjoyment not giving the least thought to what cold water or chilled drink does.

Use of cold water soon after the meals increases the chances of indigestion. It solidifies the fats in the food and also draws energy from your body to rise to body temperature. Basic purpose of drinking water is to maintain moisture level in the body. The water does so whether cold or hot. If it is warm, it will perform the same function without causing problems. Apart from the logic, it has been proved even scientifically that taking cold water after the meals is harmful for the heart, stomach and general health.

Normal temperature of our body is 37 degrees Celsius, which is equivalent to 98.6 degrees Fahrenheit. At this temperature the body function is optimum. More than this is considered as fever while less than this reduces the working efficiency by inducing general weakness. For better health, temperature inside the body must remain normal or else many troubles start brewing underneath and show up at some stage.

The benefits of drinking warm water are not restricted to just heart and stomach. It is the whole body that benefits. Developing this habit would take some time but try it for few weeks and feel the results. Remember that your health primarily depends on your dietary habits, on what you eat and drink.

It is strongly recommended that one should not take a full glass of water immediately after the meal. A glassful will not let the stomach do what it should and rather hinder correct digestion. Generally, one quarter to half a glass of warm water should be enough. After an hour or two, you can drink as much as you like but not cold water. Warm it up before you take.

3.3. FOOD GROUPS

Grains, the largest food group in many nutrition guides, include oats, barley and bread. Cookies, however, are categorized as sugars.

Vegetables, the second largest food group in many nutrition guides, come in a wide variety of shapes, colors and sizes.

A food group is a collection of foods that share similar nutritional properties or biological classifications. Nutrition guides typically divide foods into food groups and recommend daily servings of each group for a healthy diet. In the United States for instance, in conflict of interest and under the influence of the food industry it is supposed to promote, over time USDA has described food as being in from 4 to 11 different groups.

The Most Common Food Groups

- Dairy, also called milk products and sometimes categorized with milk alternatives or meat, is typically a smaller category in nutrition guides. Examples of dairy products include milk, butter, ghee, yogurt, cheese, cream and ice cream, is typically a very small category in nutrition guides, if present at all, and is sometimes listed apart from other food groups. The categorization of dairy as a food group with recommended daily servings has been criticized by, for example, the Harvard School of Public Health. The HSPH points out that "research has shown little benefit, and considerable potential for harm, of such high dairy intakes. Moderate consumption of milk or other dairy products—one to two servings a day are fine, and likely have some benefits for children. But it's not essential for adults, for a host of reasons."

- Fruits, sometimes categorized with vegetables, include apples, oranges, bananas, berries and lemons. Fruits are carbohydrates, like sugar, dairy, grains, and starches.

- Grains, beans and legumes; grains are also called cereals and sometimes inclusive of potatoes and other starches, is often the largest category in nutrition guides. Examples include wheat, rice, oats, barley, bread and pasta. An example of beans would be baked beans and soy beans, while an example of legumes would be lentils and chickpeas.

- Meat, sometimes labeled protein and occasionally inclusive of legumes, eggs, meat analogues and/or dairy, is typically a medium- to smaller-sized category in nutrition guides. Examples include chicken, fish, turkey, pork and beef.

- Confections also called sugary foods and sometimes categorized with fats and oils, are typically a very small category in nutrition guides, if present at all, and is sometimes listed apart from other food groups. Examples include candy, soft drinks, and chocolate.

- Vegetables, sometimes categorized with fruit and occasionally inclusive of legumes, are typically a large category second only to grains, or sometimes equal or superior to grains, in nutrition guides. Examples include spinach, carrots, onions, peppers, and broccoli.

- Water is treated in very different ways by different food guides. Some exclude the category, others list it separately from other food groups, and yet others make it the center or foundation of the guide. Water is sometimes categorized with tea, fruit juice, vegetable juice and even soup, and is typically recommended in plentiful amounts.

Uncommon Food Groups

- The number of "common" food groups varies depending on who is defining them. Canada's Food Guide, which has been in continual publication since 1942 and is the second most requested government document (after the income tax form) in Canada, recognizes only four official food groups, listing the remainder of foods as "another." Some of these "others" include:

- Alcohol is listed apart from other food groups and recommended only for certain people in moderation by Harvard's Healthy Eating Pyramid and the University of Michigan's Healing Foods Pyramid, while Italy's food pyramid includes a half-serving of wine and beer.

3.4. DIET AND DIABETES

Making healthy food choices can lower your risk of developing diabetes or its complications. But some diseases can be silent predators, offering few or no warning signs to alert you early on that help is needed. One such disease is diabetes. The incidence of diabetes mellitus is increasing so quickly that it has become a global epidemic.

3.4.1. WHAT IS DIABETES?

As food is digested, it is broken down into glucose (also known as sugar), which provides energy and powers our cells. Insulin, a hormone made in the pancreas, moves the glucose from the blood to the cells. However, if there is not enough insulin or the insulin is not working properly, then the glucose stays in the blood and causes blood sugar levels to rise. Excess body fat can be a major factor in type 2 diabetes. Experts believe that fat accumulated in the belly and waist may indicate a higher risk for diabetes. More specifically, fat in the pancreas and the liver appear to disrupt the body's regulation of blood sugar.

There are three main types of diabetes: type 1, type 2, and gestational diabetes. Type1 results from the pancreas no longer being able to make insulin and is usually found in children, teens, and young adults. Gestational diabetes can occur near the end of a woman's pregnancy and usually disappears after the baby's birth.

The most common form of diabetes is type 2. Risk factors include being overweight; not getting enough physical activity; having a parent or sibling with diabetes; being African-American, Asian-American, Latino, Native American, or Pacific Islander; being a woman who had gestational diabetes or gave birth to a baby who weighed more than nine pounds; having high blood pressure, having low levels of High-density lipoproteins, HDL (good cholesterol) or high triglycerides; and having pre-diabetes.

Diabetes: Why Is It Dangerous

"When poorly controlled diabetes causes blood glucose levels that are too high or too low, you may not feel well," explains Claudia L. Morrison, RD, outpatient diabetes program coordinator at Washington Hospital Center in Washington, D.C. "Diabetes that is poorly controlled over time can lead to complications that affect the body from head to toe." Issues can occur with everything from one's eyes, kidneys, and nerves to reproductive organs, blood vessels, and gums. But the most serious problems are heart disease and risk of stroke.

Diabetes: What Role Does Diet Play

"Food can either promote diabetes or help prevent it, depending on how it affects the body's ability to process glucose," says Elizabeth Ricanati, MD, medical director of the Cleveland Clinic's Lifestyle 180 Program in Cleveland. "People should avoid foods that increase blood sugar and those that raise cholesterol, such as processed foods, foods high in saturated fats or with trans fats, and foods with added sugars and syrups."

Processed foods as well as items high in fat or sugar not only can disrupt the balance between glucose and insulin, resulting in inflammation, but can also contribute to risk factors such as being overweight.

Carbohydrates too, need to be watched. While they are necessary to fuel the body, some carbohydrates raise blood glucose levels more than others. "The glycemic index (GI) measures how a carbohydrate-containing food raises blood glucose". "Foods are ranked based on how they compare to a reference food such as white bread. Dry beans and legumes, all non-starchy vegetables, and many whole-grain breads and cereals all have a low GI."

Diabetes: What Is a Healthy Diet?

A healthy diet for diabetes is virtually the same as a healthy diet for anyone. Eat reasonably sized portions to avoid gaining weight, and include fruits and vegetables (limit juice to no more than eight ounces a day); whole grains rather than processed ones; fish and lean cuts of meat; beans and legumes; and liquid oils. Limit saturated fats and high-calorie snacks and desserts like chips, cake, and ice cream, and stay away from trans fats altogether.

Thirty minutes of exercise most days of the week and losing 5 to 10 percent of body weight, if a person is overweight, are also crucial in reducing the risk of type 2 diabetes.

Finally, anyone experiencing frequent urination, extreme thirst or hunger, unexplained weight loss, fatigue, blurry vision, or frequent infections should see a doctor for a blood test to check for diabetes. With careful attention and healthy lifestyle choices, diabetes can be kept under control.

Three Steps That May Reduce the Risk of Diabetes

1. **Have your level of blood sugar tested if you are in a high-risk group**. A medical disorder known as prediabetes—a condition in which blood sugar is moderately higher than normal—often precedes type 2 diabetes. Both conditions are unhealthy, but there is a difference: Although diabetes can be controlled, it cannot yet be cured. On the other hand, some prediabetics have been able to bring their blood sugar back to normal levels. Prediabetes may have no obvious symptoms. Hence, this condition may go unnoticed.

   Prediabetes is not harmless, however. Besides being a precursor to type2 diabetes, it has recently been linked to an increased risk of dementia. If you are overweight, not physically active, or have a family history of diabetes, you might already have prediabetes. A blood test can tell you if you do.

2. **Choose healthful food**. You might benefit from doing the following whenever it is possible and practical: Eat smaller portions than usual. Instead of sugary fruit juice and carbonated beverages, drink water, tea, or coffee. Eat whole-grain bread, rice, and pasta in moderation rather than refined foods. Eat leaner meats, fish, nuts, and beans.

3. **Stay physically active.** Exercise can lower your blood sugar and help you maintain a healthy weight. Swap some TV time for exercise time, recommends one expert.

   You cannot change your genes, but you can change your lifestyle. Doing what we can to improve our health is worth the effort.

3.5. NUTRITION

3.5.1. NUTRITION GUIDELINES

With so many diets and quick weight-loss promises on the market today, it's hard to remember what a healthy diet really looks like. Start here with the basics of good nutrition.

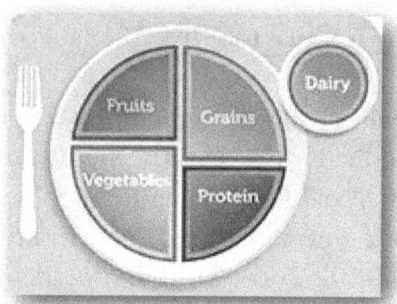

Figure 3.1: Diet Plate

Diet pills, fad diets, foods to boycott, foods to eat exclusively. With all the crazy diet advice out there, do you even remember the basics of healthy eating? Get rid of the clutter when it comes to diets, and use basic good nutrition guidelines and the **U.S. Department of Agriculture (USDA)'s MyPlate** as your framework for healthy eating.

Human nutrition refers to the provision of essential nutrients necessary to support life and health. Generally, people can survive up to 40 days without food, a period largely depending on the amount of water consumed, stored body fat, muscle mass and genetic factors.

Poor nutrition is a chronic problem often linked to poverty, poor nutrition understanding and practices, and deficient sanitation and food security. Malnutrition globally provides many challenges to individuals and societies. Lack of proper nutrition contributes to worse class performance, lower test scores, and eventually less successful students and a less productive and competitive economy. Malnutrition and its consequences are immense contributors to deaths and disabilities worldwide. Promoting good nutrition helps children grow, promotes human development and advances economic growth and eradication of poverty.

3.5.2. FOOD GROUPS AND HEALTHY NUTRITION

So how do we know what healthy meals should look like? The USDA is responsible for publishing nutritional guidelines for healthy eating based on ongoing research. Although the basics have not really changed, recently, there have been a few adjustments.

The major adjustment is the focus on filling half of your plate with fruits and vegetables at every meal. Women need at least seven servings of fruits and vegetables each day, while men need at least nine. Carbohydrates are also an important part of a healthy diet, contrary to many popular fad diets being touted today — the key is consuming fiber-rich complex carbohydrates like beans, whole grains, and fruit.

3.5.3. FOOD GROUPS AND HEALTHY NUTRITION: USDA RECOMMENDATIONS

Here are details about the USDA's recommended nutritional guidelines to follow for a healthy eating plan:

- Focus on fruits and vegetables: Fill half of your plate with fruits and vegetables at every meal.
- Go for low-fat dairy: Consume at least three cups of low-fat or fat-free milk each day or the equivalent in cheese, yogurt, or other calcium-rich foods.
- Choose whole grains: Get at least six to eight servings of whole grains each day. Grains should fill a quarter of your plate at each meal.
- Steer clear of trans and saturated fats, sodium (salt), sugars, and cholesterol: Limit fat to only about 20 to 35 percent of total calorie intake and avoid trans and saturated fats.
- Choose lean proteins: Fill the remaining quarter of your plate with lean protein. About 15 percent of your total calories should come from proteins, such as skin, fish, beans, nuts, and legumes.

3.5.4. FOOD GROUPS AND HEALTHY NUTRITION: GUIDELINES TO GET YOU GOING

Here are some other tips to help you develop a healthy eating plan. If you keep these general nutrition rules in mind, you'll be on the right track toward healthy eating for life:

- Pay attention to portion control; quantities depend on whether you're trying to lose or maintain weight. In most restaurants, an appetizer serving is often closer to an appropriate serving size than an entrée.
- Always drink plenty of water.
- Vary your food choices to make sure you get a wide variety of vitamins and other nutrients and to avoid boredom.
- Know the recommended daily calorie intake for your age, weight, height, activity level, and gender.
- Do not deprive yourself of foods you love; just enjoy them in moderation.

Start thinking about the basics of diet and nutrition again, and make nutritional guidelines part of your everyday life. It won't be a diet, it won't be a fad, and it definitely won't be temporary. It will be your new healthy lifestyle, and when you think, "What's for dinner?" the answer will naturally be a healthy choice.

3.5.5. WHY FRUITS AND VEGETABLES ARE VITAL

Eating a diet rich in fruits and vegetables is important for good health. Find out why experts say Mother Nature's bounty packs better nutrients than supplements.

If we are what we eat, then many of us must be tripping all over the place due to a lack of balance. The Department of Health and Human Services (HHS) and the U.S. Department of Agriculture's (USDA) new guidelines state that we should be eating 5 to 13 servings of nature's best, depending on the number of calories you need.

Fruits and vegetables may prevent many illnesses. Eating fruits and vegetables may reduce your risk of cardiovascular diseases, stroke, type 2 diabetes, and even some forms of cancer. Recent studies revealed that the more fruits and vegetables people ate daily, the less chance they would develop cardiovascular diseases.

The relationship between fruits and vegetables and cancer prevention has been more difficult to prove. However, recent studies show that some types of produce are associated with lower rates of some types of cancer. For example, the World Cancer Research Fund and the American Institute for Cancer Research suggest that mouth, stomach, and colorectal cancers are less likely with high intakes of non-starchy foods like leafy greens, broccoli, and cabbage. Though studies have been mixed, lycopene, a carotenoid that gives tomatoes their red color, may help stave off prostate cancer.

Fruits and vegetables are great for watching your weight. They are low in fat and calories, and loaded with fiber and water, which create a feeling of fullness. This is particularly helpful for dieters who want more filling calories. Plus, that fiber helps keep you "regular."

Fruits and vegetables: get your fill

Remember that variety is the spice of life when adding fruits and vegetables to your diet. It is important to eat produce of various colors because each fruit or vegetable offers a different nutrient — think of it as nutritional cross-training. Trying new foods can be exciting, and be sure to sample every color in the produce rainbow.

The right number of servings of fruits and vegetables for you all depends on your daily caloric intake needs. A good way to find out how many servings you should be eating is by eating a fruit or vegetable at every meal and snack.

Do not let season, accessibility, or cost affect your fruit- and vegetable-friendly diet. If finding fresh produce is difficult, choose frozen, canned (low-sodium), or dried varieties. Also, 100 percent juice counts toward your servings, though it does not offer the full fiber of whole fruit.

The power of prevention may lie in a salad bowl or a plate of fruit. When we take advantage of produce, our bodies return the favor by reducing our risk of developing various illnesses.

3.6. MALNUTRITION

Malnutrition refers to insufficient, excessive, or imbalanced consumption of nutrients. In developed countries, the diseases of malnutrition are most often associated with nutritional imbalances or excessive consumption. Although there are more people in the world who are malnourished due to excessive consumption, according to the United Nations World Health Organization, the real challenge in developing nations today, more than starvation, is combating insufficient nutrition – the lack of nutrients necessary for the growth and maintenance of vital functions.

The causes of malnutrition are directly linked to inadequate macronutrient consumption and disease, and are indirectly linked to factors like "household food security, maternal and child care, health services, and the environment."

Table 3.3: Individual nutrition challenges

Nutrients	Deficiency	Excess
Food Energy	starvation, marasmus	obesity, diabetes mellitus, cardiovascular disease
Simple carbohydrates	None	diabetes mellitus, obesity
Complex carbohydrates	None	obesity
Saturated fat	low sex hormone levels	cardiovascular disease
Trans fat	None	cardiovascular disease
Unsaturated fat	None	obesity
Fat	malabsorption of fat-soluble vitamins, rabbit starvation (if protein intake is high), during development: stunted brain development and reduced brain weight.	cardiovascular disease
Omega-3 fats	cardiovascular disease	bleeding, hemorrhages
Omega-6 fats	None	cardiovascular disease, cancer
Cholesterol	during development: deficiencies in myelinization of the brain	cardiovascular disease
Protein	kwashiorkor	
Sodium	hyponatremia	hypernatremia, hypertension
Iron	anemia	cirrhosis, cardiovascular disease
Iodine	goiter, hypothyroidism	Iodine toxicity (goiter, hypothyroidism)
Vitamin A	xerophthalmia and night blindness, low testosterone levels	hypervitaminosis A (cirrhosis, hair loss)
Vitamin B₁	beriberi	
Vitamin B₂	cracking of skin and corneal unclearation	
Niacin	pellagra	dyspepsia, cardiac arrhythmias, birth defects
Vitamin B₁₂	pernicious anemia	
Vitamin C	scurvy	diarrhea causing dehydration
Vitamin D	rickets, osteoporosis, balance, immune system, inflammation	hypervitaminosis D (dehydration, vomiting, constipation)
Vitamin E	nervous disorders	hypervitaminosis E (anticoagulant excessive bleeding)
Vitamin K	hemorrhage	
Calcium	osteoporosis, tetany, carpopedal spasm, laryngospasm, cardiac arrhythmias	fatigue, depression, confusion, anorexia, nausea, vomiting, constipation, pancreatitis, increased urination
Magnesium	hypertension	weakness, nausea, vomiting, impaired breathing, and hypotension
Potassium	hypokalemia, cardiac arrhythmias	hyperkalemia, palpitations

CHAPTER 4

EXERCISE AND SEDENTARY LIFESTYLE

4.1. PHYSICAL EXERCISE

WANT TO FEEL better, have more energy and perhaps even live longer? Look no further than exercise. The health benefits of regular exercise and physical activity are hard to ignore. And the benefits of exercise are yours for the taking, regardless of your age, sex or physical ability.

Physical exercise is any bodily activity that enhances or maintains physical fitness and overall health and wellness. It is performed for various reasons, including strengthening muscles and the cardiovascular system, honing athletic skills, weight loss or maintenance, and merely enjoyment. Frequent and regular physical exercise boosts the immune system and helps prevent the "diseases of affluence" such as heart disease, cardiovascular disease, Type 2 diabetes, and obesity. It may also help prevent depression, help to promote or maintain positive self-esteem, improve mental health generally, and can augment an individual's sex appeal or body image, which has been found to be linked with higher levels of self-esteem. Childhood obesity is a growing global concern, and physical exercise may help decrease some of the effects of childhood and adult obesity. Health care providers often call exercise the "miracle" or "wonder" drug—alluding to the wide variety of proven benefits that it can provide.

"There is no drug in current or prospective use that holds as much promise for sustained health as a lifetime program of physical exercise." Dr. Walter Bortz II

4.1.1. CLASSIFICATION

Physical exercises are generally grouped into three types, depending on the overall effect they have on the human body:

- Aerobic exercise is any physical activity that uses large muscle groups and causes your body to use more oxygen than it would while resting. The goal of aerobic exercise is to increase cardiovascular endurance. Examples of aerobic exercise include cycling, swimming, brisk walking, skipping rope, rowing, hiking, playing tennis, continuous training, and long slow distance training.

- Anaerobic exercise is also called Strength or Resistance training and can firm, strengthen, and tone your muscles, as well as improve bone strength, balance, and coordination. Examples of strength moves are pushups, lunges, and bicep curls using dumbbells. Anaerobic exercise also includes weight training, functional training, eccentric training, and interval training, sprinting and high-intensity interval training increase short-term muscle strength.

- Flexibility exercises stretch and lengthen your muscles. Activities such as stretching help to improve joint flexibility and keep muscles limber. The goal is to improve the range of motion which can reduce the chance of injury.

Physical exercise can also include training that focuses on accuracy, agility, power, and speed.

Sometimes the terms 'dynamic' and 'static' are used. 'Dynamic' exercises such as steady running tend to produce a lowering of the diastolic blood pressure during exercise, due to the improved blood flow. Conversely, static exercise (such as weight-lifting) can cause the systolic pressure to rise significantly (during the exercise).

There are three broad Intensities of exercise
Light exercise
The exerciser is able to talk while exercising. Going for a walk is an example of light exercise.

Moderate exercise
The exerciser feels slightly out of breath during the session. Examples could be walking briskly, cycling moderately, or walking up a hill. Scientists from Lawrence Berkeley National Laboratory, Life Science Division in Berkeley, California reported in the journal Arteriosclerosis, Thrombosis and Vascular Biology that brisk walking is as effective as running in reducing a person's risk of hypertension (high blood pressure), high cholesterol and diabetes.

Vigorous exercise
The exerciser is panting during the activity. The exerciser feels a body push much nearer its limit, compared to the other two intensities. This could include running, cycling fast, and heavy weight training.

4.2. HEALTH BENEFITS AND EFFECTS OF EXERCISE

Physical exercise is important for maintaining physical fitness and can contribute positively to maintaining a healthy weight, building and maintaining healthy bone density, muscle strength, and joint mobility, promoting physiological well-being, reducing surgical risks, and strengthening the immune system. Developing research has demonstrated that many of the benefits of exercise are mediated through the role of skeletal muscle as an endocrine organ. That is, contracting muscles release multiple substances known as myokines which promote the growth of new tissue, tissue repair, and multiple anti-inflammatory functions, which in turn reduce the risk of developing various inflammatory diseases.

Exercise controls weight

Exercise can help prevent excess weight gain or help maintain weight loss. When you engage in physical activity, you burn calories. The more intense the activity, the more calories you burn. You do not need to set aside large chunks of time for exercise to reap weight-loss benefits. If you cannot do an actual workout, get more active throughout the day in simple ways — by taking the stairs instead of the elevator or revving up your household chores.

Exercise combats health conditions and diseases

Worried about heart disease? Hoping to prevent high blood pressure? No matter what your current weight, being active boosts high-density lipoprotein (HDL), or "good," cholesterol and decreases unhealthy triglycerides. This one-two punch keeps your blood flowing smoothly, which decreases your risk of cardiovascular diseases. In fact, regular physical activity can help you prevent or manage a wide range of health problems and concerns, including stroke, metabolic syndrome, type 2 diabetes, depression, and certain types of cancer, arthritis and falls. Cardiovascular system

The beneficial effect of exercise on the cardiovascular system is well documented. There is a direct relation between physical inactivity and cardiovascular mortality, and physical inactivity is an independent risk factor for the development of coronary artery disease. There is a dose-response relation between the amount of exercise performed from approximately 700 to 2000 kcal of energy expenditure per week and all-cause mortality and cardiovascular disease mortality in middle-aged and elderly populations. The greatest potential for reduced mortality is in the sedentary who become moderately active. Most beneficial effects of physical activity on cardiovascular disease mortality can be attained through moderate-intensity activity (40% to 60% of maximal oxygen uptake, depending on age). Persons who modify their behavior after myocardial infarction to include regular exercise have improved rates of survival. Persons who remain sedentary have the highest risk for all-cause and cardiovascular disease mortality.

Exercise boosts immune system

Although there have been hundreds of studies on exercise and the immune system, there is little direct evidence on its connection to illness. Epidemiological evidence suggests that moderate exercise has a beneficial effect on the human immune system. Moderate exercise has been associated with a 29% decreased incidence of upper respiratory tract infections (URTI), but studies of marathon runners found that their prolonged high-intensity exercise was associated with an increased risk of infection occurrence. However, another study did not find the effect. Immune cell functions are impaired following acute sessions of prolonged, high-intensity exercise, and some studies have found that athletes are at a higher risk for infections. The immune systems of athletes and nonathletes are generally similar. Athletes may have slightly elevated natural killer cell count and cytolytic action, but these are unlikely to be clinically significant.

Vitamin C supplementation has been associated with lower incidence of URTIs in marathon runners.

Biomarkers of inflammation such as C-reactive protein, which are associated with chronic diseases, are reduced in active individuals relative to sedentary individuals, and the positive effects of exercise may be due to its anti-inflammatory effects. In individuals with heart disease, exercise interventions lower blood levels of fibrinogen and C-reactive protein, an important cardiovascular risk marker. The depression in the immune system following acute bouts of exercise may be one of the mechanisms for this anti-inflammatory effect.

Exercise improves brain function

Physical activity has been shown to be neuroprotective in many neurodegenerative and neuromuscular diseases. Evidence suggests that it reduces the risk of developing dementia. A 2008 review of cognitive enrichment therapies (strategies to slow or reverse cognitive decline) concluded that "physical activity and aerobic exercise in particular, enhances older adults' cognitive function".

There are several possibilities for why exercise is beneficial for the brain. Examples are as follows:

- increasing the blood and oxygen flow to the brain;
- increasing growth factors that help neurogenesis and promote synaptic plasticity- possibly improving short and long term memory;
- increasing chemicals in the brain that help cognition, such as dopamine, glutamate, norepinephrine, and serotonin.

Physical activity is thought to have other beneficial effects related to cognition as it increases levels of nerve growth factors, which support the survival and growth of a number of neuronal cells.

Exercise boosts energy
Winded by grocery shopping or household chores? Regular physical activity can improve your muscle strength and boost your endurance. Exercise and physical activity deliver oxygen and nutrients to your tissues and help your cardiovascular system work more efficiently. And when your heart and lungs work more efficiently, you have more energy to go about your daily chores.

Exercise improves mood
Need an emotional lift? Or need to blow off some steam after a stressful day? A workout at the gym or a brisk 30-minute walk can help. Physical activity stimulates various brain chemicals that may leave you feeling happier and more relaxed. You may also feel better about your appearance and yourself when you exercise regularly, which can boost your confidence and improve your self-esteem.

A number of factors may contribute to depression including being overweight, low self-esteem, stress, and anxiety. Endorphins act as a natural pain reliever and antidepressant in the body. Endorphins have long been regarded as responsible for what is known as "runner's high", a euphoric feeling a person receives from intense physical exertion. However, recent research indicates that anandamide may possibly play a greater role than endorphins in "runner's high". When a person exercises, levels of both circulating serotonin and endorphins are increased. These levels are known to stay elevated even several days after exercise is discontinued, possibly contributing to improvement in mood, increased self-esteem, and weight management. Exercise alone is a potential prevention method and/or treatment for mild forms of depression. Research has also shown that when exercise is done in the presence of other people (familiar or not), it can be more effective in reducing stress than simply exercising alone.

Exercise promotes better sleep
Struggling to fall asleep or to stay asleep? Regular physical activity can help you fall asleep faster and deepen your sleep. Just do not exercise too close to bedtime, or you may be too energized to fall asleep.

Exercise puts the spark back into your sex life
Do you feel too tired or too out of shape to enjoy physical intimacy? Regular physical activity can leave you feeling energized and looking better, which may have a positive effect on your sex life. But there's more to it than that. Regular physical activity can lead to enhanced arousal for women. And men who exercise regularly are less likely to have problems with erectile dysfunction than are men who do not exercise.

Exercise can be fun
Exercise and physical activity can be a fun way to spend some time. It gives you a chance to unwind, enjoy the outdoors or simply engage in activities that make you happy. Physical activity can also help you connect with family or friends in a fun social setting. So, take a dance class, hit the hiking trails or join a soccer team. Find a physical activity you enjoy, and just do it. If you get bored, try something new.

The bottom line on exercise

Exercise and physical activity are a great way to feel better, gain health benefits and have fun. As a general goal, aim for at least 30 minutes of physical activity every day. If you want to lose weight or meet specific fitness goals, you may need to exercise more. Remember to check with your doctor before starting a new exercise program, especially if you have not exercised for a long time, have chronic health problems, such as heart disease, diabetes or arthritis, or you have any concerns.

4.3. EXCESSIVE EXERCISE

Too much exercise can be harmful. Without proper rest, the chance of stroke or other circulation problems increases, and muscle tissue may develop slowly. Extremely intense, long-term cardiovascular exercise, as can be seen in athletes who train for multiple marathons, has been associated with scarring of the heart and heart rhythm abnormalities.

Inappropriate exercise can do more harm than good, with the definition of "inappropriate" varying according to the individual. For many activities, especially running and cycling, there are significant injuries that occur with poorly regimented exercise schedules. Injuries from accidents also remain a major concern, whereas the effects of increased exposure to air pollution seem only a minor concern.

In extreme instances, over-exercising induces serious performance loss. Unaccustomed overexertion of muscles leads to rhabdomyolysis (damage to muscle) most often seen in new army recruits. Another danger is overtraining, in which the intensity or volume of training exceeds the body's capacity to recover between bouts.

Stopping excessive exercise suddenly may create a change in mood. Feelings of depression and agitation can occur when withdrawal from the natural endorphins produced by exercise occurs. Exercise should be controlled by each body's inherent limitations. While one set of joints and muscles may have the tolerance to withstand multiple marathons, another body may be damaged by 20 minutes of light jogging.

This must be determined for each individual. Too much exercise may cause a woman to miss her period, a symptom known as amenorrhea.

4.4. WHAT IS A SEDENTARY LIFE-STYLE?

How do you know if you are active enough? There are various opinions on what constitutes a sedentary life-style. However, most health experts agree on general guidelines that apply to most people. One explanation used by several health organizations is that you are sedentary if you:

- Do not exercise or engage in some vigorous activity for at least 30 minutes three times a week.
- Do not move from place to place while engaging in leisure activities.
- Rarely walk more than 100 yards during the course of a day.
- Remain seated most of your waking hours.
- Have a job that requires little physical activity.

Are you getting enough exercise? If not, you can start doing something about it today. 'But I just don't have the time,' you may say. When you get up in the morning, you are simply too tired. At the start of the day, you hardly have enough time to get yourself ready and get to your job. Then, after a long day, again you feel too tired to exercise and have too many other things to do.

Or perhaps you are among the many that start to exercise but quit after just a few days because they find it too strenuous, perhaps even feeling sick after exercising. Others shy away from exercise because they think that a good fitness program must include grueling routines of weight lifting, lengthy daily runs covering many miles, and carefully choreographed stretching sessions.

And then there is the expense and the perceived inconvenience. Joggers need suitable clothing and shoes. For strength training you need weights or special exercise machines. A sports-club membership can be costly. Travel to the gym can be time-consuming. Still, none of the above need prevent you from leading a physically active life and reaping the health benefits.

Set realistic goals
First of all, if you plan to start an exercise program, do not set unrealistic goals. Start slowly, and work your way up. Scientists have recently acknowledged the value of light-to-moderate physical activity, and they recommend that sedentary people increase their activity gradually. For instance, the UC Berkeley Wellness Letter, a newsletter on nutrition, fitness, and stress management published by the University of California, advises: "Start by adding a few minutes of increased activity to your day, and work up to 30 minutes most, and preferably all, days of the week." The newsletter explains that "all you have to do are the normal things, like walking and taking the stairs, but just more often, a little longer, and/or a little faster."

Beginners should focus on regularity rather than intensity. Once your strength and endurance have improved, you can work on increasing the intensity of the exercise. This can be done by incorporating longer sessions of more vigorous activity, such as brisk walking, jogging, stair climbing, or cycling. Eventually for a more well-rounded fitness program, you may even include some weight lifting and some stretching exercises. Many health experts, however, no longer subscribe to the "no pain, no gain" approach to exercise. So, to reduce the risk of injury and to avoid the burnout and discouragement that often lead to quitting, keep exercise at a comfortable level.

Be regular
Those who never seem to have time for physical activity would welcome a recommendation made by the Wellness Letter. It explains that "short bouts of exercise during the course of a day have an additive benefit. That is, three 10-minute periods of exertion can be almost as beneficial as one 30-minute session." Thus, you do not need to engage in lengthy periods of vigorous exercise in order to reap substantial health

benefits. The Journal of the American Medical Association reports that researchers have found that "light to moderate activity, as well as vigorous activity, was associated with a lower risk of experiencing coronary heart disease."

But regularity is a must. With that in mind, you may want to look at your calendar and schedule specific dates and times for exercise. After a few weeks of a sustained exercise program, you will likely find that it has become a normal part of your life. Once you begin to enjoy the health benefits, you may actually look forward to your sessions of physical activity.

4.4.1. AN ACTIVE LIFE IS A BETTER LIFE

While it is true that as little as 30 minutes of daily physical activity can have a positive impact on your health, according to the latest medical advice, more is better. It is now recommended that to maintain a maximal level of cardiovascular health, you should accumulate up to 60 minutes of physical activity every day. Again, this can be achieved by engaging in several brief sessions spread throughout the day.

The bottom line is that your body is designed to move around and engage in regular physical activity. A sedentary life-style is harmful to your health. And there is no vitamin, medicine, food, or surgical procedure that can replace your need to remain active. Also, we must all face the fact that an adequate exercise routine, whether moderate or vigorous, whether done in short installments or longer sessions, requires time. Just as you make the time for eating and sleeping, it is vital that you also make the time to remain physically active. This involves self-discipline and good personal organization.

There is no hassle-free exercise program. The inconveniences and sacrifices involved in maintaining an active life-style however, pale into insignificance when compared with the life-threatening dangers of an inactive life-style. Stay active, break a sweat now and again, work those muscles—you might live a healthier and longer life!

4.4.2. A HIGHER LEVEL OF EXERTION

While a moderate increase in everyday physical activities can bring significant health benefits, researchers say that greater results are obtained with more vigorous exercise. Below are some options.

Health professionals recommend consulting a doctor before embarking on a program of vigorous exercise.

- **Brisk walking:** Sometimes called speed walking or power walking, this is one of the more convenient ways to exercise. All you need is a comfortable pair of walking shoes and a path. Walk with a longer stride and a pace that is considerably faster than a leisurely stroll. Try to reach a speed of about three to five miles (4 to 9 kilometers) an hour.

- **Jogging:** When you jog, you are basically running at a slow pace. Jogging has been described as the most efficient way to achieve cardiovascular fitness. However, because of its higher impact, jogging is more likely to cause muscle and joint injury. Hence, joggers are reminded about the need for adequate shoes, stretching, and moderation.

- **Bicycling:** If you have a bicycle, you can enjoy a very effective form of exercise. Bicycling can burn up to 700 calories an hour. Like walking and jogging, however, bicycling is often done on the streets. For this reason you must remain alert as you ride, taking all the necessary precautions to prevent accidents.

- **Swimming:** You can exercise all the major muscle groups in your body by swimming. It also helps keep your joints flexible, and it can give you virtually all the cardiovascular benefits of jogging. Because swimming is gentler on your body, it is often recommended for people with arthritis, back problems, or weight problems as well as for pregnant women. Avoid swimming alone!

- **Rebounding:** This aerobic exercise requires the use of a small trampoline. It simply involves bouncing on the trampoline. Proponents claim that rebounding improves both blood and lymphatic circulation, increases the capacity of the heart and lungs, and improves muscle tone, coordination, and balance.

4.4.3. LIFTING AND STRETCHING

Scientists have recently concluded that a balanced fitness program should include some form of strength training, such as weight lifting. Done properly, weight lifting not only builds muscle but also increases bone density and helps reduce body fat. Many health experts also recommend stretching to improve flexibility and blood circulation. Stretching can help your joints achieve a full range of motion.

However, to avoid injury, both weight training and stretching must be done properly. You may want to learn a few basic guidelines by reading reliable material on the subject or consulting your doctor.

4.5. EXERCISE AND MIND

Scientists have discovered that vigorous physical activity can affect a number of mood-altering brain chemicals, such as dopamine, norepinephrine, and serotonin. This might explain why there are many claims of mental well-being after exercising. Some studies even suggest that people who exercise regularly are less likely to be depressed than those who are sedentary. While some of these studies are not conclusive, many doctors recommend exercise as a method of reducing stress and anxiety.

Everyday activities that can improve your health

According to recent studies, sedentary people may benefit from simply increasing the frequency of everyday activities that require moderate levels of exertion. You may want to try some of the following.

- Climb stairs instead of taking the elevator or ride the elevator to a floor somewhat short of your destination and then take the stairs the rest of the way.
- If you use public transportation, get off a few stops early, and walk the rest of the way.

- When using your own vehicle, get in the habit of parking some distance away from your destination. In a multilevel parking garage, park on a level that will allow you to climb the stairs.
- Walk while you talk. You do not always need to be seated when having casual conversations with friends or family members.
- If you have a sedentary job, find opportunities to work in a standing position, and move around whenever possible.

4.6. DRINKING ENOUGH WATER

Inadequate water consumption during exercise can be harmful. It can cause fatigue, decreased coordination, and muscle cramping. When you exercise, you sweat at a faster rate, and this can lead to a drop in your blood volume. If you do not replenish the water that is lost through perspiration, the heart has to work harder to circulate the blood. It is suggested that to avoid dehydration, you should drink water before, during, and after an exercise session.

CHAPTER 5

SKIN CARE AND SUNSCREEN AGENTS

GOOD SKIN CARE and healthy lifestyle choices can help delay the natural aging process and prevent various skin problems.

5.1. SKIN CARE TIPS

1. Protect yourself from the sun

One of the most important ways to take care of your skin is to protect it from the sun. A lifetime of sun exposure can cause wrinkles, age spots and other skin problems as well as increase the risk of skin cancer.

For the most complete sun protection:

- **Use sunscreen.** Use a broad-spectrum sunscreen with an SPF (Sunscreen Protection Factor) of at least 15. Apply sunscreen generously, and reapply every two hours or more often if you're swimming or perspiring.
- **Seek shade.** Avoid the sun between 10 a.m. and 2 p.m., when the sun's rays are strongest.
- **Wear protective clothing.** Cover your skin with tightly woven long-sleeved shirts, long pants and wide-brimmed hats. Also consider laundry additives, which give clothing an additional layer of ultraviolet protection for a certain number of washings, or special sun-protective clothing — which is specifically designed to block ultraviolet rays.

2. Do not smoke

Smoking makes your skin look older and contributes to wrinkles. Smoking narrows the tiny blood vessels in the outermost layers of skin, which decreases blood flow. This depletes the skin of oxygen and nutrients that are important to skin health.

Smoking also damages collagen and elastin- the fibers that give your skin strength and elasticity. In addition, the repetitive facial expressions you make when smoking such as pursing your lips when inhaling and squinting your eyes to keep out smoke can contribute to wrinkles.

If you smoke, the best way to protect your skin is to quit. Ask your doctor for tips or treatments to help you stop smoking.

3. Treat your skin gently

Daily cleansing and shaving can take a toll on your skin. To keep it gentle:

- **Limit bath time.** Hot water and long showers or baths remove oils from your skin. Limit your bath or shower time, and use warm rather than hot water.
- **Avoid strong soaps.** Strong soaps and detergents can strip oil from your skin. Instead, choose mild cleansers.
- **Shave carefully.** To protect and lubricate your skin, apply shaving cream, lotion or gel before shaving. For the closest shave, use a clean, sharp razor. Shave in the direction the hair grows, not against it.
- **Pat dry.** After washing or bathing, gently pat or blot your skin dry with a towel so that some moisture remains on your skin.
- **Moisturize dry skin.** If your skin is dry, use a moisturizer that fits your skin type. For daily use, consider a moisturizer that contains SPF.

4. Eat a healthy diet

A healthy diet can help you look and feel your best. Eat plenty of fruits, vegetables, whole grains and lean proteins. The association between diet and acne is not clear — but some research suggests that a diet rich in vitamin C and low in unhealthy fats and processed or refined carbohydrates might promote younger looking skin.

5. Manage stress
Uncontrolled stress can make your skin more sensitive and trigger acne breakouts and other skin problems. To encourage healthy skin and a healthy state of mind, take steps to manage your stress. Set reasonable limits, scale back your to-do list and make time to do the things you enjoy. The results might be more dramatic than you expect.

5.2. NATURAL SKIN CARE

Natural skin care is the care of the skin using naturally derived ingredients (such as herbs, roots, essential oils and flowers) combined with naturally occurring carrier agents, preservatives, surfactants, humectants and emulsifiers (everything from natural soap to oils to pure water). The classic definition of natural skin care is based on using botanically sourced ingredients currently existing in or formed by nature, without the use of synthetic chemicals, and manufactured in such a way to preserve the integrity of the ingredients.

As a result of this definition, many people who use natural skin care products, generally make their own products at home from naturally occurring ingredients. Many people use natural skin care recipes to make remedies to care for their skin at home. Many spas and skin care salons now focus on using more naturally derived skin care products.

Some examples of natural skin care ingredients include jojoba, safflower oil, rose hip seed oil, shea butter, beeswax, witch hazel, aloe vera, tea tree oil, and chamomile. Many of these natural ingredient combinations can be tailored specifically to the individual's skin type or skin condition.

There is, however, no actual definition of natural according to the U.S. Food and Drug Administration (FDA). All ingredients are chemicals by definition. "Derived" ingredients are unnatural both according to the original substance and the method of derivation.

The term natural has considerable market value in promoting skin care cosmetic products to consumers, but dermatologists say it has very little medical meaning and the FDA states the claim has no legal meaning. Despite pressure from advocacy groups such as The Environmental Working Group (EWG) the FDA has not defined what natural is or how to achieve it.

The FDA recommends understanding the ingredient label and says: "There is no list of ingredients that can be guaranteed not to cause allergic reactions, so consumers who are prone to allergies should pay careful attention to what they use on their skin", further warning that there is no basis in fact or scientific legitimacy to the notion that products containing natural ingredients are good for the skin". Food preservatives are commonly used to preserve the safety and efficacy in these products.

Ayurvedic skin care
Ayurvedic skin care is derived from medicinal practices that began over 5,000 years ago in India. Ayurvedic medicine and healing practices are based on Indian philosophical, psychological, conventional, and medicinal understandings. Ayurvedic approach to skin care is holistic and considers the mind, body, and spirit together. Ayurvedas practices the belief that there are three basic principles or humors born out of five basic elements that exist in nature. These principles are known as Vata, Pitta, and Kapha. These principles are believed to work together in harmony to make up the entire body.

Ayurvedic skin types
In Ayurvedic skin care, there are seven different types of constitution that govern skin and hair types: Vata, Pitta, Kapha, Vata-Pitta, Vata-Kapha, Pitta-Kapha, or Vata-Pitta-Kapha. Most people fall into a combination of two of the three principles.

Ayurveda advises to modify one's diet, exercise, lifestyle and supplements according to one's constitution of these three humors. Most of the skin care products contain the following herbs—aloe vera, almond, avocado, carrot, castor, clay, cocoa, coconut oil, cornmeal, cucumber, cutch tree, emu oil, ginkgo biloba, ginseng, grape seed oil, ground almond and wallnut shell, horse chestnut, witch hazel and honey.

Egg oil skin care

Egg oil has many applications in skin care and can be used as an excipient/carrier in a variety of cosmetic preparations such as creams, ointments, sun-screen products or lotions where it acts as an emollient, moisturizer, anti-oxidant, penetration enhancer, occlusive skin conditioner and anti-bacterial agent. As an occlusive agent, it protects against dehydration without disturbing the pores and is easily incorporated in topical preparations since it forms stable oil in water emulsions.

Honey skin care

Honey's natural antioxidant and anti-microbial properties and ability to absorb and retain moisture have been recognized and used extensively in skin care treatments as they help to protect the skin from the damage of the sun's rays and rejuvenate depleted skin. Honey is also often used to treat acne, either dabbed directly on spots or as a face mask, and has been used successfully to treat diabetic foot ulcers. It also fixes scars and marks on the skin.

Shea butter skin care

Shea butter is derived from the kernel of the shea tree (Vitellaria paradoxa). The nuts are then crushed, boiled and manipulated in order to extract a light colored fat, which is commonly referred to as shea butter. Pure shea butter resembles lumps of hard caramel ice cream. Being edible, shea butter is often used in food preparations, but it has gained huge popularity in the western world due to its widespread use in several beauty products such as lotions, cosmetics, shampoos, conditioners and many more. Shea butter is known for its cosmetic properties as a moisturizer and emollient.

The main components of shea butter include oleic acid, stearic acid, linoleic acid and others. It gets absorbed quickly into the skin as it melts at body temperature. Shea butter may be refined or unrefined. Raw or unrefined shea butter is the purest form of shea butter which is most natural and least processed. Since it is extracted manually, it is able to retain its vitamins, minerals and other natural properties. Refined shea butter, on the other hand, is the processed form of butter.

Shea butter exhibits several health benefits particularly for the skin and hair. It is used in a variety of cosmetics and medicinal formulas in combination with other botanical ingredients. Some of the health benefits of shea butter are given below.

- **Healing Qualities:** Shea butter is known for its healing properties, which can be attributed to the presence of several fatty acids and plant sterols such as oleic, palmitic, stearic and linolenic acids. These oil-soluble components do not undergo saponification or convert into soap on coming in contact with alkali. Shea butter is more non-saponifiable than other nut oils and fats, thus imparting it a great healing potential for the skin. Raw unrefined shea butter is effective for curing skin rashes, skin peeling after tanning, scars, stretch marks, frost bites, burns, athletes foot, insect bites and stings, arthritis and muscle fatigue.
- **Antioxidant Qualities:** Shea butter contains plant antioxidants such as vitamins A and E, as well as catechins. The vitamins A and E protect the cells from free radicals and environmental damage. The cinnamic acid esters in shea fat helps in preventing skin damage from ultraviolet radiation.
- **Anti-inflammatory Properties:** Several derivatives of cinnamic acid are found in shea butter which exhibit anti-inflammatory properties. Research has proved that in addition to its anti-inflammatory benefits, lupeol cinnamate found in shea butter prevents the development of tumors. Its anti-inflammatory properties render it beneficial for improvement of skin conditions.
- **Sun Protection:** Shea butter acts as a natural sunscreen by providing protection against the ultraviolet radiations of sun though the level of protection offered may be variable. Shea butter is considered as the best skincare for winter and after-sun

care as it provides the extra moisture, nutrients and protection needed by your skin during the cold season and summer.

- **Healing Agent:** Shea butter has amazing healing properties. It is often used as a base in medicinal ointments due to its anti-inflammatory properties. It has been used since ages for the treatment of scars, eczema, blemishes, skin discolorations, chapped lips, stretch marks, dark spots and in reducing the irritation caused by psoriasis. Due to its high content of vitamin A, it is effective in promoting healing and disinfection; and soothes skin allergies like poison ivy and insect bites. Vitamin E acts as a rejuvenator for soothing and healing rough and chapped skin.

- **Anti-ageing Benefits:** Shea Butter is considered as one of the best anti-ageing and moisturizing agents for skin. It stimulates the production of collagen, the youthful scaffolding protein in the skin. The vitamins A and E found in this butter keep the skin supple, nourished and radiant and prevent premature wrinkles and facial lines. Shea butter penetrates the skin easily without clogging the pores and is effective for dry skin.

- **Baby Care:** Shea butter is an excellent natural moisturizer which is devoid of chemicals. Thus, it is ideal for baby care as besides being gentle and soft on skin, it is specially adapted for delicate and sensitive skin of babies. It can be for after bath application on skin and as also for healing eczema or diaper rash on the skin of babies.

- **Lip Care:** Shea butter is easily absorbable and provides extra moisture and nutrients that are needed during cold season and dry weather. Thus, it acts as a perfect lip balm to protect your lips from cold and dry weather and is effective for treating dry and chapped lips.

- **Restores Skin Elasticity:** Non-saponifiable matter and vitamin E in this butter are vital ingredients for maintaining skin-elasticity. Thus, application of shea butter restores the elasticity of the skin and helps maintain an even skin-tone besides hydrating, softening and beautifying it.

- **Soothes Dry and Irritated Scalp:** Shea butter is effective in soothing a dry itchy scalp or dandruff. It possesses anti-inflammatory qualities and gets absorbed into the skin without leaving a greasy residue or clogging the pores. Being rich in vitamins A and E, it soothes dryness, repairs breakage and mends split ends. Hence, it is extremely effective in providing relief against dry scalp, dermatitis, eczema and psoriasis.
- **Moisturizer:** The presence of vitamins A and E makes shea butter an excellent moisturizer to moisturize your hair from roots to tips. Thus, it can be used as a natural conditioner. It is highly effective in locking in moisture without leaving the hair greasy or heavy. Shea butter has wide usage in curly hair treatments due to its emollient qualities. A number of chemical treatments like straighteners, perms, curlers etc., are responsible for stripping off natural moisture from the hair. Shea butter can help restore this lost moisture.
- **Hair Protection:** Shea butter provides protection to the hair against the harmful free radicals in the air and water and harsh weather conditions. Moreover, shea butter has low amount of SPF which is sufficient enough to protect the hair from sun damage caused due to exposure to ultraviolet radiation and repairs the damage that has already been caused by harsh weather and sun. This is largely due to the fact that once absorbed, shea butter coats the hair shaft so that it is protected from a heat tool or any other damaging material being passed along the hair. This is particularly beneficial for processed or colored hair. It also protects the hair against salt and chlorine when applied before swimming.
- **Hair Softener:** Shea butter is great for softening and revitalizing damaged and brittle hair. Due to its non-greasy nature, it helps to control and spread excess oil in the scalp. Massaging the hair with generous amounts of shea butter can give soft and silky tresses. This benefit of shea butter is applicable for dry as well as fragile curly hair. Shea butter should be applied twice a week for hair growth, improving hair texture and moisturizing the hair.

Jojoba skin care

Jojoba is used for skin care because it is a natural moisturizer for the skin. Jojoba is actually a liquid wax that becomes solid below room temperature, but is known as oil.

Algae skin care

Polysaccharides derived from algae (the singular is alga) are natural moisturizers and can be used in cosmetics as humectants. Because they are marine organisms, seaweeds and other types of marine algae are high in trace elements, including copper, iodine, iron, magnesium, manganese, phosphorus, potassium and zinc. Marine algae are also well-known for being rich in vitamins, particularly A, B1, B2, B3, B5, B12, C, D, E and K. Other constituents – they vary from species to species – moisturize, promote the strengthening of skin tissue, particularly elastin and collagen, and balancing the moisture barrier in skin cells so that the tissues remain hydrated. In particular, marine algae are renowned for containing natural ingredients which provide antioxidant protection.

5.3. SUNSCREEN PROTECTION

Although the sun is necessary for life, too much sun exposure can lead to adverse health effects, including skin cancer. It is estimated that 90 percent of non-melanoma skin cancers and 65 percent of melanoma skin cancers are associated with exposure to ultraviolet (UV) radiation from the sun.

By themselves, sunscreens might not be effective in protecting you from the most dangerous forms of skin cancer. However, sunscreen use is an important part of your sun protection program. Used properly, certain sunscreens help protect human skin from some of the sun's damaging UV radiation. But according to recent surveys, most people are confused about the proper use and effectiveness of sunscreens.

5.3.1. HOW UV RADIATION AFFECTS SKIN AND RISKS

UV radiation, a known carcinogen, can have a number of harmful effects on the skin. The two types of UV radiation that can affect the skin are UVA and UVB. Both have been linked to skin cancer and a weakening of the immune system. They also contribute to premature aging of the skin and cataracts (a condition that impairs eyesight), and cause skin color changes.

UVA Rays

UVA rays, which are not absorbed by the ozone layer, penetrate deep into the skin and heavily contribute to premature aging. Up to 90 percent of the visible skin changes commonly attributed to aging are caused by sun exposure.

UVB Rays

These powerful rays, which are partially absorbed by the ozone layer, mostly affect the surface of the skin and are the primary cause of sunburn. Because of the thinning of the ozone layer, the effects of UVB radiation will pose an increased threat.

5.3.2. SOME PEOPLE ARE PREDISPOSED TO ADVERSE HEALTH EFFECTS

Everybody, regardless of race or ethnicity, is subject to the potential adverse effects of overexposure to the sun. However, some people are more vulnerable than others to the harmful effects of the sun.

Skin Type

Skin type affects the degree to which some people burn and the time it takes them to burn. The Food and Drug Administration (FDA) classifies skin type on a scale from 1 to 6. Individuals with lower number skin types (1 and 2) have fair skin and tend to burn rapidly and more severely. Individuals with higher number skin types (5 and 6), though capable of burning, have darker skin and do not burn easily.

5.3.3. HOW SUNSCREENS WORK AND WHAT IS THE SUN PROTECTION FACTOR (SPF)

Sunscreens protect your skin by absorbing and/or reflecting UVA and UVB rays. The FDA requires that all sunscreens contain a Sun Protection Factor (SPF) label. The SPF reveals the relative amount of sunburn protection that a sunscreen can provide an average user (tested on skin types 1, 2, and 3) when correctly used.

Sunscreens with an SPF of at least 15 are recommended. You should be aware that an SPF of 30 is not twice as protective as an SPF of 15; rather, when properly used, an SPF of 15 protects the skin from 93 percent of UVB radiation, and an SPF 30 sunscreen provides about 97 percent protection.

Although the SPF ratings found on sunscreen packages apply mainly to UVB rays, many sunscreen manufacturers include ingredients that protect the skin from some UVA rays as well. **These "broad-spectrum" sunscreens are highly recommended.**

5.3.4. EFFECTS OF SUN EXPOSURE

The same people who are most likely to burn are also most vulnerable to skin cancer. Studies have shown that individuals with large numbers of freckles and moles also have a higher risk of developing skin cancer. Although people with higher-number skin types have a lower incidence of skin cancer, they should still take action to protect their skin and eyes from overexposure to the sun, since cases of skin cancer in people with darker skin are often not detected until later stages when it is more dangerous.

Additional factors

Certain diseases, such as lupus, can also make a person more sensitive to sun exposure. Some medications, such as antibiotics and antihistamines and even certain herbal remedies, can cause extra sensitivity to the sun's rays. Discuss these issues with your physician.

5.3.5. WHAT ARE THE ACTIVE INGREDIENTS IN SUNSCREEN?

Chemical Ingredients

Broad-spectrum sunscreens often contain a number of chemical ingredients that absorb UVA and UVB radiation. Many sunscreens contain UVA-absorbing **avobenzone** or a **benzophenone** (such as dioxybenzone, oxybenzone, or sulisobenzone), in addition to UVB-absorbing chemical ingredients (some of which also contribute to UVA protection). In rare cases, chemical ingredients cause skin reactions, including acne, burning, blisters, dryness, itching, rash, redness, stinging, swelling, and tightening of the skin. Consult a physician if these symptoms occur. These reactions are most commonly associated with para-aminobenzoic acid (PABA)-based sunscreens and those containing benzophenones. Some sunscreens also contain alcohol, fragrances, or preservatives, and should be avoided if you have skin allergies.

Physical Ingredients

The physical compounds titanium dioxide and zinc oxide reflect, scatter, and absorb both UVA and UVB rays. These ingredients, produced through chemical processes, do not typically cause allergic reactions. Using new technology, the particle sizes of zinc oxide and titanium dioxide have been reduced, making them more transparent without losing their ability to screen UV.

5.3.6. HOW DO I APPLY SUNSCREEN?

Use a broad-spectrum sunscreen with an SPF rating of 15 or higher. Apply sunscreen 20 minutes before going out into the sun (or as directed by the manufacturer) to give it time to absorb into your skin. Apply it generously and regularly— about 1 ounce every 2 hours—and more often if you are swimming or perspiring. A small tube containing between 3 and 5 ounces of sunscreen might only be enough for one person during a day at the beach.

Do not forget about lips, ears, feet, hands, bald spots and the back of the neck. In addition, apply sunscreen to areas under bathing suit straps, necklaces, bracelets, and sunglasses. Keep sunscreen until the expiration date or for no more than 3 years, because the sunscreen ingredients might become less effective over time.

According to the FDA, "water resistant" sunscreens must maintain their SPF after 40 minutes of water immersion, while "very water resistant" sunscreens must maintain their SPF after 80 minutes of water immersion. Either type of water-resistant sunscreen must be reapplied regularly, as heavy perspiration, water, and towel drying remove the sunscreen's protective layer.

How Can I Maximize My Sun Protection?

Because the active sunscreen ingredients will not usually block out the complete spectrum of UVA and UVB rays, sunscreens by themselves might not offer enough protection to prevent skin cancer and some of the other sun-related ailments. To thoroughly protect yourself, you should take as many of the following action steps as you can:

- *Do Not Burn*
- *Avoid Sun Tanning and Tanning Beds*
- *Generously Apply Sunscreen*
- *Wear Protective Clothing*
- *Seek Shade*
- *Use Extra Caution near Water, Snow, and Sand*
- *Watch for the UV Index*
- *Get Vitamin D Safely*

5.4. TATTOO HEALTH RISKS

Tattoos are everywhere—or so it seems. Rock stars, sports figures, fashion models, and movie stars flaunt them. Many teenagers have followed suit, proudly displaying tattoos on their shoulders, hands, waists, and ankles.

The *World Book Encyclopedia* says, "Tattooing is the practice of making permanent designs on the body. It is done by pricking small holes in the skin with a sharpened stick, bone, or needle that has been dipped in pigments with natural colors."

5.4.1. HEALTH RISKS

There are also health concerns you should consider. What you are doing is breaking the skin and introducing pigmented material into the area. Even though the needle only goes in a little way, anytime you break the skin, you have a risk of bacterial or viral infection. Once pigment is in, even if there is no infection, there is always the chance of contact allergies, dermatitis and allergic reactions that can cause skin to get red, swollen, crusty and itchy.

Despite the intended permanence of tattoos, various methods are used in attempts to remove them: Laser removal (burning the tattoo away), surgical removal (cutting the tattoo away), dermabrasion (sanding the skin with a wire brush to remove the epidermis and dermis), salabrasion (using a salt solution to soak the tattooed skin), and scarification (removing the tattoo with an acid solution and creating a scar in its place). These methods are expensive and can be painful. *"It is more painful to have a tattoo removed by laser than to get the original tattoo," says Teen magazine.*

Like all fads, tattoos may lose their appeal over time. Really, is there any garment—whether a pair of jeans, a shirt, a dress, or a pair of shoes—that you love so much that you would commit to wearing it for the rest of your life? Of course not! Styles, cuts, and colors change. Unlike a piece of clothing, however, tattoos are hard to shed. Besides, what is "cool" to you when you are 16 might not be very appealing when you are 30.

Think before you ink. Don't make a decision that you may regret!

5.5. SKIN CANCER

Skin cancers are cancers that arise from the skin. They are due to the development of abnormal cells that have the ability to invade or spread to other parts of the body. There are three main types: basal cell cancer (BCC), squamous cell cancer (SCC) and melanoma. *The first two together along with a number of less common skin cancers are known as nonmelanoma skin cancer (NMSC).* Basal cell cancer grows slowly and can damage the tissue around it but is unlikely to spread to distant areas or result in death. It often appears as a painless raised area of skin that may be shiny with small blood vessel running over it or may present as a raised area with an ulcer. Squamous cell cancer is more likely to spread. It usually presents as a hard lump with a scaly top but may also form an ulcer. Melanomas are the most aggressive. Signs include a mole that has changed in size, shape, color, has irregular edges, has more than one color, is itchy or bleeds.

Greater than 90% of cases are caused by exposure to ultraviolet radiation from the sun. This exposure increases the risk of all three main types of skin cancer. Exposure has increased partly due to a thinner ozone layer. Tanning beds are becoming another common source of ultraviolet radiation. For melanomas and basal cell cancers, exposure during childhood is particularly harmful. For squamous cell cancers total exposure, irrespective of when it occurs, is more important. Between 20% and 30% of melanomas develop from moles. People with light skin are at higher risk as are those with poor immune function such as from medications or HIV/AIDS. *Diagnosis is by biopsy.*

Decreasing exposure to ultraviolet radiation and the use of sunscreen appears to be effective methods of preventing melanoma and squamous cell cancer. It is not clear if sunscreen affects the risk of basal cell cancer. Nonmelanoma skin cancer is usually curable. Treatment is generally by surgical removal but may less commonly involve radiation therapy or topical medications such as fluorouracil. Treatment of melanoma may involve some combination of surgery, chemotherapy, radiation therapy, and targeted therapy. In those people whose disease has spread to other areas of their bodies, palliative care may be used to improve quality of life. Melanoma has one of the higher survival rates among cancers, with over 86% of people in the UK and more than 90% in the United States surviving more than 5 years.

Skin cancer is the most common form of cancer, globally accounting for at least 40% of cases. It is especially common among people with light skin. The most common type is nonmelanoma skin cancer, which occurs in at least 2-3 million people per year. This is a rough estimate, however, as good statistics are not kept. About 80% are basal cell cancers in nonmelanoma skin cancers and 20% squamous cell cancers. Basal cell and squamous cell cancers rarely result in death. Globally in 2012 melanoma occurred in 232,000 people, and resulted in 55,000 deaths. Australia and New Zealand have the highest rates of melanoma in the world. The three main types of skin cancer have become more common in the last 20 to 40 years, especially in those areas which mostly are Caucasian. Check out World Health Organization (WHO) reports.

CHAPTER 6

STRESS AND COPING WITH STRESS

STRESS IS A state of mental or emotional strain or tension resulting from adverse or demanding circumstances. It is your body's way of responding to any kind of demand. It can be caused by both good and bad experiences. It is important to figure out what causes stress for you. Everyone feels and responds to stress differently. Tracking your stress may help. Get a notebook, and write down when something makes you feel stressed. Then write how you reacted and what you did to deal with the stress. Tracking your stress can help you find out what is causing your stress and how much stress you feel. Then you can take steps to reduce the stress or handle it better.

To get stress under control:

- Find out what is causing stress in your life.
- Look for ways to reduce the amount of stress in your life.
- Learn healthy ways to relieve stress and reduce its harmful effects.

6.1. IDENTIFY THE SOURCES OF STRESS IN YOUR LIFE

Stress management starts with identifying the sources of stress in your life. This is not as easy as it sounds. Your true sources of stress are not always obvious, and it is all too easy to overlook your own stress-inducing thoughts, feelings, and behaviors. Sure, you may know that you are constantly worried about work deadlines. But maybe it is your procrastination, rather than the actual job demands, that leads to deadline stress.

To identify your true sources of stress, look closely at your habits, attitude, and excuses:

- Do you explain away stress as temporary ("I just have a million things going on right now") even though you cannot remember the last time you took a breather?
- Do you define stress as an integral part of your work or home life ("Things are always crazy around here") or as a part of your personality ("I have a lot of nervous energy, that's all").
- Do you blame your stress on other people or outside events, or view it as entirely normal and unexceptional?

Until you accept responsibility for the role you play in creating or maintaining it, your stress level will remain outside your control.

6.2. START A STRESS JOURNAL

A stress journal can help you identify the regular stressors in your life and the way you deal with them. Each time you feel stressed; keep track of it in your journal. As you keep a daily log, you will begin to see patterns and common themes. Write down:

- What caused your stress (make a guess if you are unsure)
- How you felt, both physically and emotionally
- How you acted in response
- What you did to make yourself feel better
- Look at how you currently cope with stress

Think about the ways you currently manage and cope with stress in your life. Your stress journal can help you identify them. Are your coping strategies healthy or unhealthy, helpful or unproductive? Unfortunately, many people cope with stress in ways that compound the problem.

Unhealthy ways of coping with stress
These coping strategies may temporarily reduce stress, but they cause more damage in the long run:

- Smoking
- Drinking too much
- Overeating or under eating
- Zoning out for hours in front of the TV or computer
- Withdrawing from friends, family, and activities
- Using pills or drugs to relax
- Sleeping too much
- Procrastinating
- Filling up every minute of the day to avoid facing problems
- Taking out your stress on others (lashing out, angry outbursts, physical violence)

Learning healthier ways to manage stress
If your methods of coping with stress aren't contributing to your greater emotional and physical health, it is time to find healthier ones. There are many healthy ways to manage and cope with stress, but they all require change. You can either change the situation or change your reaction. When deciding which option to choose, it is helpful to think of the four As: avoid, alter, adapt, or accept.

Since everyone has a unique response to stress, there is no "one size fits all" solution to managing it. No single method works for everyone or in every situation, so experiment with different techniques and strategies. Focus on what makes you feel calm and in control.

6.3. DEALING WITH STRESSFUL SITUATIONS: THE FOUR A'S
Change the situation:

- Avoid the stressor
- Alter the stressor

Change your reaction:

- Adapt to the stressor
- Accept the stressor

6.4. STRESS MANAGEMENT STRATEGY

It may seem that there is nothing you can do about stress. The bills will not stop coming, there will never be more hours in the day and your career and family responsibilities will always be demanding. But you have more control than you might think. The simple realization that you are in control of your life is the foundation of stress management. Managing stress is all about taking charge: of your thoughts, emotions, schedule, and the way you deal with problems.

6.4.1. AVOID UNNECESSARY STRESS

Not all stress can be avoided, and it is not healthy to avoid a situation that needs to be addressed. You may be surprised, however, by the number of stressors in your life that you can eliminate.

Learn how to say "no" – Know your limits and stick to them. Whether in your personal or professional life, taking on more than you can handle is a surefire recipe for stress.

Avoid people who stress you out – If someone consistently causes stress in your life and you cannot turn the relationship around, limit the amount of time you spend with that person or end the relationship entirely.

Take control of your environment – If the evening news makes you anxious, turn the TV off. If traffic's got you tense, take a longer but less-traveled route. If going to the market is an unpleasant chore, do your grocery shopping online.

Avoid hot-button topics – If you get upset over religion or politics, cross them off your conversation list. If you argue repeatedly about the same subject with the same people; excuse yourself or stop bringing it up when it is the topic of discussion.

Pare down your to-do list – Analyze your schedule, responsibilities, and daily tasks. If you have got too much on your plate, distinguish between the "shoulds" and the "musts." Drop tasks that are not truly necessary to the bottom of the list or eliminate them entirely.

6.4.2. ALTER THE SITUATION

If you cannot avoid a stressful situation, try to alter it. Figure out what you can do to change things so the problem does not present itself in the future. Often, this involves changing the way you communicate and operate in your daily life.

Express your feelings instead of bottling them up. If something or someone is bothering you, communicate your concerns in an open and respectful way. If you do not voice your feelings, resentment will build and the situation will likely remain the same.

Be willing to compromise. When you ask someone to change their behavior, be willing to do the same. If you both are willing to bend at least a little, you will have a good chance of finding a happy middle ground.

Be more assertive. Do not take a backseat in your own life. Deal with problems head on, doing your best to anticipate and prevent them. If you have got an exam to study for and your chatty roommate just got home, say upfront that you only have five minutes to talk.

Manage your time better. Poor time management can cause a lot of stress. When you are stretched too thin and running behind, it is hard to stay calm and focused. But if you plan ahead and make sure you do not overextend yourself, you can alter the amount of stress you are under.

6.4.3. ADAPT TO THE STRESSOR

If you cannot change the stressor, change yourself. You can adapt to stressful situations and regain your sense of control by changing your expectations and attitude.

Reframe problems. Try to view stressful situations from a more positive perspective. Rather than fuming about a traffic jam, look at it as an opportunity to pause and regroup, listen to your favorite radio station, or enjoy some alone time.

Look at the big picture. Take perspective of the stressful situation. Ask yourself how important it will be in the long run. Will it matter in a month? A year? Is it really worth getting upset over? If the answer is no, focus your time and energy elsewhere.

Adjust your standards. Perfectionism is a major source of avoidable stress. Stop setting yourself up for failure by demanding perfection. Set reasonable standards for yourself and others, and learn to be okay with "good enough."

Focus on the positive. When stress is getting you down, take a moment to reflect on all the things you appreciate in your life, including your own positive qualities and gifts. This simple strategy can help you keep things in perspective.

Adjusting your attitude

How you think can have a profound effect on your emotional and physical well-being. Each time you think a negative thought about yourself, your body reacts as if it were in the throes of a tension-filled situation. If you see good things about yourself, you are more likely to feel good; the reverse is also true. Eliminate words such as "always,""never,""should," and "must." These are telltale marks of self-defeating thoughts.

6.4.4. ACCEPT THE THINGS YOU CANNOT CHANGE

Some sources of stress are unavoidable. You cannot prevent or change stressors such as the death of a loved one, a serious illness, or a national recession. In such cases, the best way to cope with stress is to accept things as they are. Acceptance may be difficult, but in the long run, it is easier than railing against a situation you can't change.

Do not try to control the uncontrollable. Many things in life are beyond our control— particularly the behavior of other people. Rather than stressing out over them, focus on the things you can control such as the way you choose to react to problems.

Look for the upside. As the saying goes, "What doesn't kill us makes us stronger." When facing major challenges, try to look at them as opportunities for personal growth. If your own poor choices contributed to a stressful situation, reflect on them and learn from your mistakes.

Share your feelings. Talk to a trusted friend face to face or make an appointment with a therapist. The simple act of expressing what you are going through can be very cathartic, even if there is nothing you can do to alter the stressful situation. Opening up is not a sign of weakness and it will not make you a burden to others. In fact, most friends will be flattered that you trust them enough to confide in them, and it will only strengthen your bond.

Learn to forgive. Accept the fact that we live in an imperfect world and that people make mistakes. Let go of anger and resentments. Free yourself from negative energy by forgiving and moving on.

6.4.5. Make time for fun and relaxation

Beyond a take-charge approach and a positive attitude, you can reduce stress in your life by nurturing yourself. If you regularly make time for fun and relaxation, you will be in a better place to handle life's stressors.

Do not get so caught up in the hustle and bustle of life that you forget to take care of your own needs. Nurturing yourself is a necessity, not a luxury.

Healthy ways to relax and recharge

- Go for a walk.
- Spend time in nature.
- Call a good friend.

- Sweat out tension with a good workout.
- Write in your journal.
- Take a long bath.
- Light scented candles.
- Savor a warm cup of coffee or tea.
- Play with a pet.
- Work in your garden.
- Get a massage.
- Curl up with a good book.
- Listen to music.
- Watch a comedy.

Set aside relaxation time. Include rest and relaxation in your daily schedule. Do not allow other obligations to encroach. This is your time to take a break from all responsibilities and recharge your batteries.

Connect with others. Spend time with positive people who enhance your life. A strong support system will buffer you from the negative effects of stress.

Do something you enjoy every day. Make time for leisure activities that bring you joy, whether it be stargazing, playing the guitar, piano, or working on your bike.

Keep your sense of humor. This includes the ability to laugh at yourself. The act of laughing helps your body fight stress in a number of ways.

6.4.6. Adopt a healthy lifestyle
You can increase your resistance to stress by strengthening your physical health.

Exercise regularly. Physical activity plays a key role in reducing and preventing the effects of stress. Make time for at least 30 minutes of exercise, three times per week. Nothing beats aerobic exercise for releasing pent-up stress and tension.

Eat a healthy diet. Well-nourished bodies are better prepared to cope with stress, so be mindful of what you eat. Start your day right with breakfast, and keep your energy up and your mind clear with balanced, nutritious meals throughout the day.

Reduce caffeine and sugar. The temporary "highs" caffeine and sugar provide often end in with a crash in mood and energy. By reducing the amount of coffee, soft drinks, chocolate, and sugar snacks in your diet, you will feel more relaxed and you will sleep better.

Avoid alcohol, cigarettes, and drugs. Self-medicating with alcohol or drugs may provide an easy escape from stress, but the relief is only temporary. Do not avoid or mask the issue at hand; deal with problems head on and with a clear mind.

Get enough sleep. Adequate sleep fuels your mind, as well as your body. Feeling tired will increase your stress because it may cause you to think irrationally.

CHAPTER 7

TOOTHACHE AND MOUTH ODOUR

7.1. TOOTHACHE: CAUSES, PREVENTIONS, SYMPTOMS AND TREATMENTS

A TOOTHACHE OR tooth pain refers to pain in and around the teeth and jaws that is usually caused by tooth decay. Toothache is a common reason for visiting the dentist. Pain from toothache can affect the teeth and jaws. Tooth decay is a common reason for toothache, which will not usually get better on its own.

Toothache pain can be constantly throbbing, or may be set off by food or drink.

7.1.1. CAUSES OF TOOTHACHE
As well as tooth decay, toothache may be caused by:

- Tooth abscess
- Tooth fracture
- A damaged filling
- Repetitive motions, such as chewing gum or grinding teeth
- Infected gums

7.1.2. TOOTHACHE PREVENTIONS
Since most toothaches are the result of tooth decay, following good oral hygiene practices can prevent them. Good oral hygiene consists of brushing regularly with fluoride-containing toothpaste, flossing once

a day, and seeing your dentist as often as advised for check-ups and dental cleaning. In addition to these practices, eat foods low in sugar and ask your dentist about sealants and fluoride applications.

7.1.3. Symptoms of toothache or pain
Symptoms of toothache may include:

- Tooth pain that may be sharp, throbbing, or constant. In some people, pain results only when pressure is applied to the tooth
- Swelling around the tooth
- Fever, headache, earache or pain upon opening your mouth wide
- Foul-tasting drainage from the infected tooth

7.1.4. Treatments for toothache
Treatment for a toothache depends on the cause. If a cavity is causing the toothache, your dentist will fill the cavity or possibly extract the tooth, if necessary. A root canal might need to be done if the cause of the toothache is found to be an infection of the tooth's nerve. Bacteria that have worked their way into the inner aspects of the tooth cause such an infection. An antibiotic may be prescribed. Phototherapy with a cold laser may also be used to reduce the pain and inflammation associated with the toothache.

Toothache remedies for pain relief
Although only a doctor can cure the source of the problem, this list of treatments and pain relief remedies should get you through the night until you can visit the dentist.

Important: If your tooth aches, there is a reason for it and it is best to have it taken care of by a professional as soon as possible instead of just treating it at home and hoping the underlying issue will go away on its own. If it is infected (gum area is swollen), do not delay in getting professional medical care.

For items that direct you to chew or for liquids that are to be swooshed around inside mouth, do so with the sore tooth and focus on surrounding area.

Do not swallow liquids, spit out when done.

- *Salt Water*: Mix a heaping spoonful of salt in a small glass of lukewarm to warm water, swoosh around inside your mouth for as long as you can, spit out. Repeat a couple times.
- *Cloves*: This is an old timer's remedy, rest a clove against the sore area until pain goes away. You can also use a drop or two of clove oil (too much can be toxic) or make a thick paste of ground cloves and water or ground cloves and olive oil.
- *Alcohol*: Swoosh a bit of whiskey, scotch, brandy or vodka. A strong mouthwash that contains alcohol will do the trick too.
- *Hydrogen Peroxide*: Swoosh a bit of hydrogen peroxide. If the taste is too horrid for you, try diluting with a bit of water.
- *Vanilla Extract*: Saturate a cotton ball with vanilla and hold in place. Can also use a cotton swab dipped in extract.
- *Almond Extract*: Same method of treatment as with Vanilla (above).
- *Peppermint Extract*: Same as with Vanilla (above).
- *Lemon Extract*: Same as with Vanilla (above).
- *Tea Tree Oil*: Just a drop or two will do the trick. You can also add some to a cotton swab and hold in place or add a few drops of tea tree oil to a small glass of lukewarm to warm water and swoosh this around.
- *Oil of Oregano*: Mix a few drops with a bit of olive oil, then saturate a cotton ball with mixture. Can replace the olive oil with lukewarm water if preferred.
- *Apple Cider Vinegar*: Soak a cotton ball with apple cider vinegar (ACV) and hold it in place. Can also try regular household vinegar.

- **Ginger Root**: Take a fresh piece of ginger and chew it a bit.
- **Garlic**: Take a clove of garlic, smash it and apply (settle it inside cheek). You can also mash some garlic with salt.
- **Peppermint Leaves**: Chew on fresh peppermint leaves. You can also use dried leaves, just hold them in place.
- **Potato**: Cut a fresh piece of potato (raw, skin off) and hold in place. Can also pound a piece of raw potato, mix in a bit of salt and use the mash.
- **Lime**: Cut a slice or wedge of lime and apply, bite into it if you can to release some of the juice. If you are sensitive to cold, first bring the lime to room temperature if it was refrigerated.
- **Onion**: Slice a piece of fresh onion and hold it inside your mouth. The onion needs to be freshly cut (so it provides a bit of onion juice).
- **Cucumber**: Slice a fresh piece of cucumber and hold it over the sore area. If refrigerated, you might want to bring the cucumber to room temperature before using (if sensitive to cold) otherwise a cool piece can be soothing. You can also mash a piece with a bit of salt.
- **Plantain**: Chew up a fresh plantain leaf. If you are too sore to chew, use the other side of your mouth. Once the leaf is macerated a bit apply it to the problem area and hold in place.
- **Cayenne Pepper**: Make a paste with cayenne pepper and water.
- **Black Pepper**: You can use this full strength or make a mix of pepper and salt.
- **Baking Soda**: Take a cotton swab and moisten it with a bit of water, dip it in baking soda (coat the swab really well with baking soda), then apply. You can also make a mouth rinse by mixing a heaping spoonful of baking soda in a small glass of lukewarm to warm water, dissolve the soda then swish the mixture in your mouth.
- **Tea**: Make a fresh cup of tea then take the used tea bag (still warm) and stick it in your mouth. Careful not to tear the bag.

The tannins that are naturally in tea leaves can help numb things.

- **_Ice Pack_**: Cover an ice pack with a face cloth or towel then hold over your cheek where the problem is. This will help numb things. If that does not work, try the opposite–a hot compress (not too hot that it burns your skin).

7.2. MOUTH ODOUR OR BAD BREATH

Many people (of all ages) have mouth odour or bad breath (also known as halitosis or malodor). Sometimes it is only for a short period, and with others it is persistent (always). It is estimated that up to 50% of people have smelly mouth all the time. You can develop halitosis even if you brush and floss regularly – in fact, in most cases, bad breath is caused by the gums and tongue – not the teeth! Bad breath is one thing that you might not notice yourself, and no one finds it easy to tell you. People will avoid you, and you can lose friends easily. It is therefore important that you look out for yourself every morning before you step out... and yes, look out for your good friends too!

7.2.1. WHAT CAUSES MOUTH ODOUR OR BAD BREATH?

Bad breath can have several causes. Most people's mouth does not smell fresh when they wake up from bed. This is normal. If you brush your teeth before going to bed, the early morning smelly mouth will not be too bad; in fact some people do not smell at all.

In most cases, bad breath is caused by bacteria in the mouth breaking down bits of food.

Persistent bad breath is often a sign of gum disease. Eating strongly flavoured foods, such as onions and garlic, can cause your breath to smell unpleasant.

Smoking and drinking a lot of alcohol can also cause bad breath.

Occasionally, bad breath is the result of an infection or illness, or taking some kinds of medication.

What to do

- Good oral hygiene is usually enough to prevent and treat bad breath. When you brush your teeth, try to brush the back of your tongue, where it is harder to reach.
- Your dentist can advise you on how to improve your oral health and can refer you for further investigation if they think there may be another cause for your bad breath.

How to find out if you have mouth odour or bad breath

- Get a very good friend to be absolutely honest, but do make sure they are a true friend.
- A simple test you can do yourself is to lick the inside of your wrist and wait for the saliva to dry. If the area you licked smells unpleasant, it is likely that your breath does too.

How to prevent bad breath or mouth odour

Bad breath can be super embarrassing, when you come back from lunch and suddenly you are breathing toxic air all over people. There are things to do and to avoid that will help you prevent bad breath and will help you cover it up if you do have it.

Brush properly and more often: Brushing your teeth properly is one of the best things you can do in your fight against bad breath. Brush at least twice a day, for at least 2 minutes and make sure to cover all the areas in your mouth. Especially focus on where the teeth meet the gum.

- Use a soft bristled brush and replace it once every 3-4 months.
- Brush either right before you eat or 1 hour afterwards (otherwise you might damage or erode the enamel of your teeth).
- Make sure to brush your tongue, because your tongue gets a lot of build-up of bacteria which can cause bad breath. Brush from the back to the front of your tongue and be certain to get the

sides, as well. You should not do more than 4 brushes on your tongue and make sure that you do not go too far back.

Floss your teeth: Flossing is another huge component to good mouth health, which includes preventing bad breath. Flossing removes the plaque and bacteria build-up from between your teeth, which even the best toothbrushes, cannot get rid of. Do this at least once a day.

- When you are flossing, focus on where the tooth meets the gum, so make sure that you scrape one way against the tooth and then against the next tooth.

Eat certain foods: There are some foods that you should be eating if you are looking to get rid of and prevent bad breath. Of course, most of these are the fruits and veggies that your parents always made you eat, but there are others as well.

- Try eating sugar-free yogurt once a day. Yogurt with good bacteria (probiotic bacteria) prevents bad breath by reducing the levels of bad breath causing sulfide compounds.
- Stock up on vitamin-D rich foods like salmon, orange juice or eggs, since vitamin-D helps reduce bad breath.
- Various herbs and spices might be linked to reducing bad breath, as well, because of their chlorophyll, although this is not entirely certain. Try adding cloves, anise, and fennel seeds to your diet.

Avoid certain foods: Eating certain foods (like garlic or onions, or anything spicy) can make your breath bad simply because they get into your bloodstream and eventually into your lungs, but there are other foods that cause bad breath, too, and that are more prevalent in Western diets.

- Avoid sugary foods and drinks. If you need a snack, grab an apple or some protein rather than a candy bar. Ensure you always drink your juice with straw to reduce contact with your teeth.

- Avoid acidic drinks. These are bad both for your breath and for the health of your teeth, as acidic drinks can hurt the enamel on your teeth. Avoid sodas as much as possible and if you have to drink them, make sure to drink them quickly without holding them in your mouth.
- Avoid coffee and alcohol. Both of these drinks provide an environment in your mouth for bacteria growth, which causes bad breath. They also dry out your mouth, which causes the bacteria to linger.

Avoid smoking or chewing tobacco: While there are many reasons to avoid or quit smoking or chewing tobacco (like cancer), bad breath is certainly one of them. The chemicals from the tar and nicotine build up in your mouth and throat and it dries out your mouth so that the bacteria remain in your mouth and throat for longer.

- A tobacco habit can also lead to gum disease, which among other more serious things, causes bad breath.

Drink lots of water: One problem that can cause bad breath or make bad breath worse is having a dry mouth. Water is odor-free and helps to flush out the food that bacteria love. It also helps promote saliva which cleanses the mouth and eliminates the stink-causing substances in food.

- Do not use coffee, sodas, or alcohol to cleanse your mouth. They will not help prevent bad breath and, in many causes, are actually the causes of your bad breath.
- Avoid drinking cold water during meals.

Use sugar-free gum or mints: Like water, sugar-free gums or mints can help speed up the production of saliva in your mouth and help flush out the bad bacteria. They can also cover up bad breath for a short period of time.

- Make sure that you are using sugar-free gum and mints, though, because sugars can help feed the bad bacteria, which will make your bad breath worse or maintain it at the same level once the gum or mint is gone.

Try mouthwash: Mouthwash is another way to deal with the immediate effects of bad breath. This will only provide you with a temporary mask for the bad breath, but that can be enough to get away from people.

- An antiseptic mouthwash will kill the bad bacteria, so if you get that it will help do more than just mask the bad odor. Look for mouthwashes with cetylpyridinium chloride, chlorine dioxide, zinc chloride and triclosan, as these kill bacteria.
- Avoid using a chlorhexidine-containing mouthwash long-term as this can stain your teeth (although this is reversible). Also, do not give mouthwash to children, especially if they are likely to swallow it.
- Try not to use mouthwashes with alcohol, especially if you are a kid, it makes your mouth very dry.

Get regular dental check-ups: Going to the dentist is actually super important to maintaining your oral health, which will help prevent and manage your bad breath. Your dentist will notice if your bad breath is caused by something more serious than simply food or drink, or not having brushed properly.

- If you have a lot of bad breath issues and you are following a strict healthy mouth regime (with brushing and eating properly), then you should definitely make an appointment to see your dentist.

Brushing your teeth and scraping your tongue before bedtime is a great way to get a head start on the bacteria that accumulate in your mouth overnight and during naps. Keeping well-hydrated while sleeping also helps a lot. Drink water one hour after meal, and avoid drinking cold drinks during meals.

Caution: Do not over-brush! This can damage your gums, which may exacerbate any existing hygiene problems. Rely on fresh water more often than your toothbrush, and switch to soft bristles if necessary. Don't assume that others like the smell of whatever it is you use to cover up a breath problem. Good hygiene is always better than nasty breath mixed with another odor, pleasant or not. Substances that you think smell nice can act as a vehicle to carry your bad breath further into others' breathing space, and others may not think such substances smell good anyway. Always scrape your tongue from back to front, in one smooth motion, and do not start this motion too far back. Don't forget to scrape the middle, also the left and right sides of the top surface of your tongue. Four quick scrapes should be plenty, after each time you sleep. Never show up at a job interview, a party, or a date with chewing gum or candy in your mouth. Many people find these habits to be offensive, and rather than covering a bad breath problem, they will most likely make it worse.

CHAPTER 8

MOOD DISORDERS

MOOD DISORDERS AFFECT about 10% of the population. Everyone experiences "highs" and "lows" in life, but people with mood disorders experience them with greater intensity and for longer periods of time than most people.

8.1. DEPRESSION AND BIPOLAR DISORDER

We all experience changes in our mood. Sometimes we feel energetic, full of ideas, or irritable, and other times we feel sad or down. But these moods usually do not last long, and we can go about our daily lives. Depression and bipolar disorder are two mental illnesses that change the way people feel and make it hard for them to go about their daily routine.

Depression is the most common mood disorder; a person with depression feels "very low." Symptoms may include: feelings of hopelessness, changes in eating patterns, disturbed sleep, constant tiredness, an inability to have fun, and thoughts of death or suicide.

People with bipolar disorder have periods of depression and periods of feeling unusually "high" or elated. The "highs" get out of hand, and the manic person can behave in a reckless manner, sometimes to the point of financial ruin or getting in trouble with the law.

While we may think of low mood or other challenges as adult problems, they can affect people at any age. Children and teens can experience mental illnesses like depression. Sometimes it can be difficult for adults to understand how difficult children's problems can be because we look at their problems through adult eyes. But the pressures of growing up can be very hard for some children. It is important that we remind ourselves that while their problems may seem unimportant to us, they can feel overwhelming to young people. It is important to take depression in young people seriously.

Two groups of mood disorders are broadly recognized; the division is based on whether a manic or hypomanic episode has ever been present. Thus, there are depressive disorders, of which the best-known and most researched is major depressive disorder (MDD) commonly called clinical depression or major depression, and bipolar disorder (BD), formerly known as manic depression and characterized by intermittent episodes of mania or hypomania, usually interlaced with depressive episodes. However, there are also psychiatric syndromes featuring less severe depression known as dysthymic disorder (similar to but milder than MDD) and cyclothymic disorder (similar to but milder than BD). Mood disorders may also be substance-induced or occur in response to a medical condition.

Cyclothymic Disorder

Bipolar disorder causes severe, unusual shifts in mood and energy that affect your ability to do normal tasks at home, school, or work. Cyclothymic disorder is often thought of as a mild form of bipolar disorder. With cyclothymic disorder, you have low-grade high periods (hypomanias) as well as brief, fleeting periods of depression that do not last as long (less than 2 weeks at a time) as in a major depressive episode. The hypomanias in cyclothymic disorder are similar to those seen in bipolar II disorder, and do not progress to full-blown manias. For example, you may feel an exaggerated sense of productivity or power, but you do not lose connection with reality. In fact, some people feel the "highs" of cyclothymic disorder are even enjoyable. They tend to not be as disabling as they are with bipolar disorder.

Its cause is unknown, but genetics may play a role; cyclothymia is more common in people with relatives who have bipolar disorder. Symptoms usually appear in adolescence or young adulthood. But because symptoms are mild, it is often difficult to tell when cyclothymia begins.

Symptoms of Cyclothymic Disorder

A diagnosis of cyclothymic disorder may result from simply describing symptoms like these:

- Episodes that involve brief, recurrent periods of depression and, at other times, episodes of hypomania; this pattern of episodes must be present for at least 2 years.
- Symptoms that persist, creating fewer than 2 symptom-free months in a row.

The episodes of cyclothymic disorder are often somewhat unpredictable. Either depression or hypomania can last for days or weeks, interspersed with a month or two of normal moods. Or, you may have no "normal" periods in between. In some cases, cyclothymic disorder progresses to full-blown bipolar disease.

Treatment for Cyclothymic Disorder

Some people with mild symptoms of cyclothymia are able to live successful, fulfilling lives. Others find their relationships troubled by depression, impulsive actions, and strong emotions. For these people, short-term medications may bring relief. However, cyclothymic disorder may not respond as well to medications as does bipolar disorder. A combination of mood stabilizers and psychotherapy is most effective. Mood stabilizers include lithium and antiseizure drugs such as Depakote, Tegretol, or Lamictal.

Treatment for Dysthymic Disorder

Staying in a constant state of moodiness is no way to live. That is one reason to seek treatment. Another is that dysthymic disorder can also increase your risk for physical diseases. If left untreated, this mood disorder can develop into more severe depression. It can also increase your risk for attempting suicide.

Psychotherapy ("talk therapy") is generally considered the treatment of choice for dysthymic disorder, and no medicine is formally FDA-approved for its treatment. However, if psychotherapy alone is not fully helpful, a two-pronged, long-term treatment approach may then include antidepressant medication in addition to psychotherapy. Some studies show that antidepressant medications or psychotherapy can be effective for dysthymic disorder, and sometimes a combination of both may work best.

Antidepressants, such as selective-serotonin reuptake inhibitors or tricyclic antidepressants, are often used to treat dysthymic disorder. Because you may need to continue treatment for a lengthy period, it is important to consider which medications not only work well but also ideally have few side effects. You may need to try more than one medication to find the one that works best. But know that it may take several weeks or longer to take effect. Successful treatment for chronic depression often takes longer than for acute (non-chronic) depression.

Take your medications as your doctor instructs. If they are causing side effects or still not working after several weeks, discuss this with your doctor. Do not suddenly stop taking your medications.

Specific kinds of talk therapy, such as cognitive behavioral therapy (CBT), psychodynamic psychotherapy, or interpersonal therapy (IPT), are known to be effective forms of psychotherapy that treat dysthymic disorder. A structured treatment lasting for a certain period of time, CBT involves recognizing and restructuring thoughts. It can help you change your distorted thinking. IPT is also a time-limited, structured treatment. Its focus is on addressing current problems and solving interpersonal conflicts. Psychodynamic psychotherapy involves exploring unhealthy or unsatisfying patterns of behavior and motivations that you may not be consciously aware of which could lead to feelings of depression and negative expectations and life experiences.

Some studies also suggest that aerobic exercise can help with mood disorders. This is most effective when done four to six times a week. But some exercise is better than none at all. Other changes may also help, including seeking social support and finding an interesting occupation. Used for patients with seasonal affective disorder, bright-light therapy may also help some people with dysthymic disorder.

8.2. MORNING DEPRESSION (DIURNAL VARIATION OF DEPRESSIVE SYMPTOMS)

Morning depression, not to be confused with seasonal affective disorder (SAD), is also known as diurnal variation of depressive symptoms (DV) or diurnal mood variation.

Morning depression is one of the core features of melancholia found in major depressive disorder (MDD). Patients with DV typically experience a worsening of depressive symptoms in the morning as opposed to in afternoon or evening.

Causes of Morning Depression: Circadian Rhythms

Nearly every function of the human body undergoes measurable changes over the course of a 24-hour day. The rhythms of hormones such as melatonin and cortisol (which affect sleep cycles and have been well-studied) but there are a lot of other changes going on as well. The circadian rhythm, or body clock, regulates everything from heart rate to body temperature and impacts functions such as cognition, alertness, and, especially, mood.

Diurnal mood variation has been shown to be, in large part, due to weakened circadian functioning. For instance, one 1997 Harvard Medical School study found that people were more likely to be in a bad mood if they were awake when their body clock expected them to be asleep—even if they would had plenty of sleep.

109

More recent research has found that any misalignment of the body clock, sleep patterns, and the external light-dark cycle may induce mood changes, especially in people who are more susceptible to depression. Therefore, anything that helps stabilize a person's circadian rhythms including exercise, stable relationships, exposure to sunlight, maintaining regular meal times, and correctly timed medications will have a positive impact on mood.

Treatments that synchronize a person's sleep-wake cycle with his or her biological clock, such as light therapy, may help some people who are suffering with depression.

Symptoms of Morning Depression

If an individual's body clock is "out of whack," his low mood states may become chronic over time, making him believe "this is just how I am." This "absorption" of the depression into one's personality is one reason why melancholic depression is often more difficult to diagnose and treat than other types of depression.

Symptoms of morning depression may fly under the radar, so to speak, but there are some clues:

- trouble getting started in the morning or a profound lack of energy
- trouble facing simple tasks such as showering or making coffee
- slowed down physical or cognitive functioning ("thinking through a fog")
- lack of concentration or inattentiveness
- intense agitation or frustration
- lack of interest in once-pleasurable activities
- empty or "numb" feelings
- changes in appetite (usually eating more than usual)
- hypersomnia (sleeping longer than normal)

Diagnosing Morning Depression

In order to diagnose melancholic depression, a doctor or mental health professional will ask a patient about changes in sleep patterns and usually some form of the following questions:

- Are your symptoms generally worse in the morning or in the evening?
- Do you have trouble getting out of bed or getting started in the morning?
- Do your moods fluctuate dramatically during the day?
- Do you have more trouble concentrating than usual?
- Do you find pleasure in activities that you enjoy?
- Have your daily routines changed recently?
- What, if anything, improves your mood?

Treatments for Morning Depression

Melancholic depression does not respond as well to selective serotonin reuptake inhibitor (SSRI) as do some other forms of depression. Studies show, however, that serotonin–norepinephrine reuptake inhibitors (SNRIs) such as venlafaxine (Effexor) may be effective for this type of depression, as are older tricyclic antidepressants. Currently, electroconvulsive therapy (ECT) has proven to be the most effective treatment for melancholic depression.

Talk therapies, such as interpersonal, cognitive behavioral therapy, and psychotherapy, are also effective in treating melancholic depressions, especially in combination with other therapies. This may be because patients with morning depression generally identify their mood states as deriving from internal sources in contrast with others who identify outside influences when describing their symptoms.

Promising new research suggests that even small shifts in sleep patterns may affect mood states. For instance, it has been found that sleep deprivation and sleep phase advance (in which a person's sleep-wake cycle is incrementally shifted) have an antidepressant effect in some people.

Light therapies like those used for patients with SAD have also shown promise.

8.3. POSTPARTUM DEPRESSION

Bringing a new baby into the family can be challenging at the better of times, both physically and emotionally. It is natural for new parents to experience mood swings, feeling joyful one minute and depressed the next. These feelings are sometimes known as the "baby blues," and often go away soon after birth. However, some parents may experience a deep and ongoing depression that lasts much longer. This is called postpartum depression.

CHAPTER 9

GENERAL HEALTH AWARENESS TIPS

9.1. HEALTH TIPS

THESE GENERAL HEALTH tips will help you dedicate yourself to a healthy lifestyle in food dieting and nutrition, exercise and healthy tips. It has been said that "Prevention is better than cure." Some illnesses cannot be avoided. Still, there is much you can do to slow down or even prevent the onset of illness. Personal health awareness begins with small steps. These easy-to-use tips can help you make small changes in your health and fitness that can have a significant, positive impact on your overall health and wellness. These will help you take charge of your health and learn what you need to do, and when you need to do it, to keep your body running at tip-top shape.

Post-defecation clean up (Wiping your butt)

Does everyone perform this common behavior the same way? Of course not. This simple method will keep your anus fresh, clean, and happy every day. Be sure you have completed your bowel movement prior to wiping commencement; this spares you unnecessary repetition of the procedure. It is important that you remain seated for the duration of the procedure, as this ensures proper area coverage and meticulous cleansing. Start out with a decent size wad of tissue; three balled-up squares should be enough. Use moderate pressure and wipe at a cautious speed from front to back. Continue with this step, using the same size wad of tissue, until absolutely no remnants remain.

Vaginal Hygiene

Hoping that someone in your life told you early on to wipe front to back. Your vagina and butt both have bacteria living in them, all of which are important to the overall functioning of those areas, but separately. The bacteria in your vagina are not the same as the ones in your butt. While vaginas are technically self-cleaning, it's totally fine to soap off your vulva and labia (the external parts of your vagina) when you're cleaning the rest of your body. However, make sure that you are using unscented soap.

Practice Good Hygiene

There are certain times when hand washing is particularly important to protect your own health and that of others. You should wash your hands: after using the toilet; after changing diapers or helping a child to use the toilet; before and after treating a wound or a cut; before and after being with someone who is sick; before preparing, serving, or eating food; after sneezing, coughing, or blowing your nose; after touching an animal or animal waste; after handling garbage. Rub your hands together to make lather, not forgetting to clean your nails, your thumbs, the backs of your hands, and between your fingers and dry with a clean cloth or a paper towel.

Healthy Breakfast

There is no better way to start your morning than with a healthy breakfast. Don't skip breakfast. Studies show that eating a proper breakfast is one of the most positive things you can do if you are trying to lose weight. Breakfast skippers tend to gain weight. A balanced breakfast includes fresh fruit or fruit juice, vegetables, a high-fibre breakfast cereal, low-fat milk or yoghurt, whole-wheat or grains toast, and a boiled egg. Try oatmeal cooked with low-fat milk, sliced almonds and berries, or top a toaster waffle with low-fat yogurt and fruit.

Use a Safe Water Supply

Ensure that all your drinking water, including the water used for brushing teeth, making ice, washing food and dishes, or cooking-comes from a safe source, such as an adequately treated public supply or sealed bottles from a reputable firm. If there is any possibility that your piped supply has been contaminated, boil your water before use or treat it with an appropriate chemical product. When using chemicals such as chlorine or water-purifying tablets; follow the maker's directions carefully. If no water-treatment products are available, add household bleach, eight drops per gallon of water (two drops per liter), mix well, and then let the water stand for 30 minutes before using it. Handle water containers with clean hands, and do not dip your hands or fingers into water used for drinking.

Regular Exercise

Regular physical activity lowers blood pressure and helps your body control stress and weight. Start by doing what exercise you can for at least 10 minutes at a time. Children and teens should get 60 or more minutes of physical activity per day, and adults should get two hours and 30 minutes per week. You don't have to hit the gym—take a walk after dinner or play a game. Learn to do stretching exercises when you wake up. It boosts circulation and digestion, and eases back pain.

Brush up on Hygiene

Many people don't know how to brush their teeth properly. Improper brushing can cause as much damage to the teeth and gums as not brushing at all. Lots of people do not brush for long enough, do not floss and do not see a dentist regularly. Hold your toothbrush in the same way that would hold a pencil, and brush for at least two minutes. This includes brushing the teeth, the junction of the teeth and gums, the tongue and the roof of the mouth. And you don't need a fancy, angled toothbrush – just a sturdy, soft-bristled one that you replace each month.

Watch Portion Sizes

Do you know if you are eating the proper portion size? Get out the measuring cups and see how close your portions are to the recommended serving size. Using smaller plates, bowls and glasses can help you keep portions under control. Use half your plate for fruits and vegetables and the other half for grains and lean meat, poultry, seafood or beans. To complete the meal, add a glass of fat-free or low-fat milk or a serving of fat-free yogurt for dessert.

Neurobics for Mind

American researchers coined the term 'neurobics' for tasks which activate the brain's own biochemical pathways and to bring new pathways online that can help to strengthen or preserve brain circuits. Get your brains fizzing with energy. Brush your teeth with your 'other' hand, take a new route to work or choose your clothes based on sense of touch rather than sight. People with mental agility tend to have lower rates of Alzheimer's disease and age-related mental decline.

Enact Family Meal Time

Research shows that family meals promote healthier eating. Plan to eat as a family at least a few times each week. Set a regular mealtime. Turn off the TV, phones and other electronic devices to encourage mealtime talk. Get kids involved in meal planning and cooking and use this time to teach them about good nutrition.

Follow Food Safety Guidelines

The America Centers for Disease Control and Prevention estimates that roughly one in six Americans gets sick from food borne disease each year. Reduce your chances of getting sick by practicing proper hand washing. Separate raw meat, poultry and seafood from ready-to-eat foods like bread and vegetables. Use a food thermometer to make sure food is properly cooked. Refrigerate food quickly at a proper temperature to slow bacteria growth.

Get Cooking

Cooking at home can be healthy, rewarding and cost-effective. Resolve to learn some cooking and kitchen basics, like how to dice an onion or how to store herbs and spices.

Get Smelly

Garlic, onions, spring onions and leeks all contain stuff that is good for you. A study at the Child's Health Institute in Cape Town found that eating raw garlic helped fight serious childhood infections. Heat destroys these properties, so eat yours raw, wash it down with fruit juice or, if you are a sissy, have it in tablet form.

Knock One Back

A glass of red wine a day is good for you. A number of studies have found this, but a recent one found that the polyphenols (a type of antioxidant) in green tea, red wine and olives may also help protect you against breast cancer. It is thought that the antioxidants help protect you from environmental carcinogens such as passive tobacco smoke.

Bone Health

Get your daily calcium by popping a tab, chugging milk or eating yoghurt. It will keep your bones strong. Remember that your bone density declines after the age of 30. You need at least 200 milligrams daily, which you should combine with magnesium, or it simply will not be absorbed.

Healthy Snacks

Healthy snacks can sustain your energy levels between meals. Whenever possible, make your snacks, combination snacks. Choose from the MyPlate food groups: whole grains, fruits, vegetables, low-fat or fat-free dairy, lean protein or nuts. Try low-fat yogurt with fruit, whole-grain crackers with low-fat cheese, or a small portion of nuts with an apple or banana.

Get to Know Food Labels

Ever wonder about what the numbers in the Nutrition Facts panel really mean? The difference between "reduced fat" and "low fat"? Or "bad cholesterol" and "good cholesterol"? The Food and Drug Administration has strict guidelines on how food label terms can be used. Read Nutrition Facts Labels before using products.

Consult a Registered Dietitian

Whether you want to lose weight, lower your cholesterol or simply eat better, consult the experts! Registered dietitians can help you by providing sound, easy-to-follow personalized nutrition advice and put you on the path to losing weight, eating well and reducing your risk of chronic disease.

Berries for Your Belly

Blueberries, strawberries and raspberries contain plant nutrients known as anthocyanidins, which are powerful antioxidants. Blueberries rival grapes in concentrations of resveratrol – the antioxidant compound found in red wine that has assumed near mythological proportions. Resveratrol is believed to help protect against heart disease and cancer.

Curry Flavour

Hot, spicy foods containing chillies or cayenne pepper trigger endorphins, the feel-good hormones. Endorphins have a powerful, almost narcotic, effect and make you feel good after exercising. But go easy on the lamb, pork and mutton and the high-fat, creamy dishes served in many Indian restaurants.

Cut out Herbs before Surgery

Some herbal supplements – from the popular St John's Wort, Tianshi and ginkgo biloba to garlic, ginger, ginseng and feverfew – can cause increased bleeding during surgery, warn surgeons. It may be wise to stop taking all medication, including herbal supplements, at least two weeks before surgery, and inform your surgeon about your herbal use.

Eat Tomato and Apple

Tomato is a superstar in the fruit and veggie pantheon. Tomatoes contain lycopene, a powerful cancer fighter. They are also rich in vitamin C. The good news is that cooked tomatoes are also nutritious, so use them in pasta, soups and casseroles, as well as in salads. The British Thoracic Society says that tomatoes and apples can reduce your risk of asthma and chronic lung diseases. Both contain the antioxidant quercetin. To enjoy the benefits, eat five apples a week or a tomato every other day.

Eat your Stress Away

Prevent low blood sugar as it stresses you out. Eat regular and small healthy meals and keep fruit and veggies handy. Herbal teas will also soothe your frazzled nerves. Eating unrefined carbohydrates, nuts and bananas boosts the formation of serotonin, another feel-good drug. Small amounts of protein containing the amino acid tryptamine can give you a boost when stress tires you out.

Load up on Vitamin C

We need at least 90 mg of vitamin C per day and the best way to get this is by eating at least five servings of fresh fruit and vegetables every day. So hit the oranges, berries, kiwi fruits and guavas! For more details of fruits, see section on sources of vitamin C.

Regular Folic Acid Intake

Folic acid should be taken regularly by all pregnant mums and people with a low immunity to disease. Folic acid prevents spina bifida in unborn babies and can play a role in cancer prevention. It is found in green leafy vegetables, liver, fruit and bran.

Diet on Vitamin A

This vitamin and beta carotene helps to boost immunity against disease. It also assists in the healing process of diseases such as measles and is recommended by the WHO. Good natural sources of vitamin A are kidneys, liver, dairy products, green and yellow vegetables, paw-paw, mangoes, chilli pepper, red sorrel and red palm oil.

Drink Pure Water

Do not have soft drinks or energy drinks while you are exercising. Stay properly hydrated by drinking enough water during your workout (just don't overdo things, as drinking too much water can also be dangerous).

While you might need energy drinks for long-distance running, in shorter exercise sessions in the gym, your body will burn the glucose from the soft drink first, before starting to burn body fat. Same goes for eating sweets. Drink more water for our bodies depend on water to regulate temperature, transport nutrients and oxygen to cells, carry away waste products and more.

Healthy Carbohydrate Eating
Carbohydrates with a high glycaemic index (GI), such as bread, sugar, honey and grain-based food will give instant energy and accelerate your metabolism. If you are trying to burn fat, stick to beans, rice, pasta, lentils, peas, soya beans and oat bran, all of which have a low GI count.

Mindful Living
You have probably heard the old adage that life's too short to stuff a mushroom. But perhaps you should consider the opposite: that life's simply too short NOT to focus on the simple tasks. By slowing down and concentrating on basic things, you will clear your mind of everything that worries you. Really concentrate on sensations and experiences again: observe the rough texture of a strawberry's skin as you touch it, and taste the sweet-sour juice as you bite into the fruit; when your partner strokes your hand, pay careful attention to the sensation on your skin; and learn to really focus on simple tasks while doing them, whether it's flowering plants or ironing your clothes.

The Secret of Stretching
When you stretch, ease your body into position until you feel the stretch and hold it for about 25 seconds. Breathe deeply to help your body move oxygen-rich blood to those sore muscles. Do not bounce or force yourself into an uncomfortable position.

Do Your Weights Workout First
Experts say weight training should be done first, because it is a higher intensity exercise compared to cardio. Your body is better able to handle

weight training early in the workout because you are fresh and you have the energy you need to work it. Conversely, cardiovascular exercise should be the last thing you do at the gym, because it helps your body recover by increasing blood flow to the muscles, and flushing out lactic acid, which builds up in the muscles while you are weight training. It is the lactic acid that makes your muscles cramp, feel stiff and sore.

Burn Fat during Intervals

To improve your fitness quickly and lose weight, harness the joys of interval training. Set the treadmill or step machine on the interval programme, where your speed and workload varies from minute to minute. Build up gradually, every minute and return to the starting speed. Repeat this routine. Not only will it be less monotonous, but you can train for a shorter time and achieve greater results.

Your Dirtiest Foot Forward

If your ankles, knees, and hips ache from running on pavement, head for the dirt. Soft trails or graded roads are a lot easier on your joints than the hard stuff. Also, dirt surfaces tend to be uneven, forcing you to slow down a bit and focus on where to put your feet – great for agility and concentration.

Burn the Boredom, Blast the Lard

Rev up your metabolism by alternating your speed and intensity during aerobic workouts. Not only should you alternate your routine to prevent burnout or boredom, but to give your body a jolt. If you normally walk at 6.5km/h on the treadmill or take 15 minutes to walk a km, up the pace by going at 8km/h for a minute or so during your workout. Do this every five minutes or so. Each time you work out; increase your bouts of speed in small increments.

Cool Off Without a Beer

Do not eat carbohydrates for at least an hour after exercise. This will force your body to break down body fat, rather than using the food you ingest. Stick to fruit and fluids during that hour, but avoid beer.

Gym Rightly

Instead of flailing away at gym, enlist the help – even temporarily of a personal trainer. Make sure you learn to breathe properly and to do the exercises the right way. You will get more of a workout while spending less time at the gym.

Stop Fuming

Do not smoke and if you smoke already, do everything in your power to quit. Do not buy into that my granny smoked and lived-to-be-90; not even the tobacco giants believe it. Apart from the well-known risks of heart disease and cancer, orthopaedic surgeons have found that smoking accelerates bone density loss and constricts blood flow. So you could live to be a 90-year-old amputee who smells of stale tobacco smoke.

Check out the Family History

Find out your family history. You need to know if there are any inherited diseases prowling your gene pool. According to the Mayo Clinic, USA, finding out what your grandparents died of can provide useful even life-saving information about what is in store for you. And be candid, not coy: 25% of the children of alcoholics become alcoholics themselves.

Do Self-Checks

Do regular self-examinations of your breasts. Most partners are more than happy to help, not just because breast cancer is the most common cancer among women. The best time to examine your breasts is in the week after your period.

Pap smear Campaign

Have a pap smear once a year. Not on our list of favourite things, but it is vital. Cervical cancer kills 200,000 women a year and it is the most prevalent form of cancer among black women, affecting more than 30 percent. But the chances of survival are nearly 100 percent if it is detected early. Be particularly careful if you became sexually active at an early age, have had multiple sex partners or smoke.

Understand Hormones

Recent research suggests that short-term (less than five years) use of hormone replacement therapy (HRT) is not associated with an increase in the risk of breast cancer, but that using it for more than ten years might be. Breast cancer is detected earlier in women using HRT, as they are more alert to the disease than other women.

Beat the Sneezes

There are more than 240 allergens, some rare and others very common. If you are a sneezer due to pollen: close your car's windows while driving, rather switch on the internal fan (drawing in air from the outside), and avoid being outdoors between 5am and 10 am when pollen counts are at their highest. Stick to holidays in areas with low pollen counts, such as the seaside and stay away from freshly cut grass.

Doggone

If you are allergic to your cat, dog, budgie or pet piglet, stop suffering the ravages of animal dander: Install an air filter in your home. Keep your pet outside as much as possible and brush them outside of the home to remove loose hair and other allergens. Better yet, ask someone else to do so.

Asthma-Friendly Sports

Swimming is the most asthma-friendly sport of all; but cycling, canoeing, fishing, sailing and walking are also good, according to the experts. Asthma need not hinder peak performance in sport.

Deep Heat

Sun rays can burn even through thick glass, and under water. Up to 35% of UVB rays and 85% of UVA rays penetrate thick glass, while 50% of UVB rays and 75% of UVA rays penetrate a meter of water and wet cotton clothing. Which means you will need sunscreen while driving your car on holiday, and water resistant block if you are swimming.

Stay Away From Fragrant Ageing

Stay away from perfumed or flavoured suntan lotions which smell of coconut oil or orange if you want your skin to stay young. These lotions contain psoralen, which speeds up the ageing process. Rather use a fake-tan lotion. Avoid sun beds, which are as bad as the sun itself.

Sunscreen can be a Smokescreen

Sunscreen is unlikely to stop you from being sunburned, or to reduce your risk of developing skin cancer. That is because most people do not apply it properly, and stay in the sun too long. Slather on sunscreen daily and reapply it often, especially if you have been in the water. How much? At least enough to fill a shot glass.

Laugh and Cry

Having a good sob is reputed to be good for you. So is laughter, which has been shown to help heal bodies, as well as broken hearts. Studies in Japan indicate that laughter boosts the immune system and helps the body shake off allergic reactions.

Keep Preventive Care Up-to-Date

Ask your doctor what screening tests and immunizations are right for you and when they are due. Then, complete them on schedule.

It is not over till it is over

Declare it over or end relationships that no longer work for you, as you could be spending time in a dead end. Rather head for more meaning-ful things. You could be missing opportunities while you are stuck in a meaningless rut, trying to breathe life into something that is long gone.

Play Safe

Wear a bike helmet, fasten your seatbelt, obey the speed limit and use the right-size car seats for kids. Avoid driving or driving with others under the influence of alcohol or drugs. Practice safe sex if you must do it.

Strong People Go for Help

Ask for assistance. Gnashing your teeth in the dark will not get you extra brownie points. It is a sign of strength to ask for assistance and people will respect you for it. If there is a relationship problem, the one who refuses to go for help is usually the one with whom the problem lies with.

Save Steamy Scenes for the Bedroom

Showering or bathing in water that is too hot will dry out your skin and cause it to age prematurely. Warm water is much better. Apply moisturizer while your skin is still damp –it will be absorbed more easily. Adding a little olive oil to your bath will help keep your skin moisturized too.

Eye Exam

Generally you need to undergo an eye exam every two years if you wear glasses or contacts or yearly if you have diabetes or other eye problems. If you have good vision, get complete eye exam starting at age 40 every two years. The schedule will be adjusted by your eye specialist based upon your exam.

Drying off Your Skin Properly

Improve your circulation and help your lymph glands to drain by the way you towel off. Helping your lymph glands function can help prevent them becoming infected. When drying off your limbs and torso, brush towards the groin on your legs and towards the armpits on your upper body. You can do the same during gentle massage with your partner.

Sugar-coated Foods

Type 2 diabetes patients are increasing, and the incidence is increasing – with new patients getting younger. New studies show this type of diabetes is often part of a metabolic syndrome (X Syndrome), which includes high blood pressure and other risk factors for heart disease. More than 80% of type 2 diabetics die of heart disease, so make sure you control your glucose levels, and watch your blood pressure and cholesterol counts. Factor-out your sugar intake in your diets.

Rest Your Body

Stress and sex make bad bedfellows, it seems. A US survey showed that stress, kids and work are main factors to dampen libido. With the advent of technology that allows us to work from home, the lines between our jobs and our personal lives have become blurred. People work longer hours, commutes are longer and work pervades all aspects of our lives, including our sexual relationships. Put sex and intimacy on the agenda, just like everything else. Good night, sweetheart; rest heals the body and has been shown to lessen the risk of heart trouble and psychological problems.

Childish Behavior

Kids build 50% of their bone mass between ages 11-19. It is imperative kids of 9 years and over get a minimum of 4 servings of calcium-rich foods or milk products each day for healthy and strong bones.

Make Family Fitness Fun

Play music and get everyone moving around the family room. Just create Boogie Nights.

Cut Back Salt Intake

The amount of salt we need is found naturally in the foods we eat. Cut back by slowly reducing daily intake.

Write down Your Thoughts

Get to write down your thoughts for five minutes each morning or night. Research shows writing that analyzes your problems and expresses your emotions is stress-relieving.

Smile at Someone

Smile helps to remove wrinkles from your face and activates neural messaging that benefits your health and happiness. Smile at someone new today; the joy you bring is good for their heart and yours. Yes you can laugh it off but not hysterically. Just smile, it is good to your health.

Clean Your Ears

Clean your ears with extra care. Wipe the outer ear with a washcloth or tissue. Do not use bobby pins, Q-tips or sharp pointed objects to clean your ears. These objects may injure the ear canal or eardrum. Use cotton swab to clean your ears

Earwax

Earwax is the ear's mechanism for self-cleaning. If you have a build-up of wax that is blocking your hearing, see your doctor to have it removed.

Eye glasses Are Not Safety Glasses

When you are working with power tools, chemicals, or lawn mowers, do not kid yourself into believing that your ordinary glasses are all the protection your eyes need. They are not because: they do not shield a sufficiently large area; there is lots of room for debris or splashing fluids to get around your glasses and into your eyes. You might be put at greater risk of injury if shards from broken lenses fly into your eyes.

Do not sit close to TV

Sitting too close to TV will strain and harm your eyesight. Keep your eyes healthy, avoid exposure to ultraviolet (UV) light.

Regular Check for Diabetes and High Blood Pressure

Have regular physical exams to check for diabetes and high blood pressure. If left untreated, these diseases can cause eye problems. In particular, diabetes and high blood pressure can lead to conditions such as diabetic retinopathy, macular degeneration, glaucoma and ocular hypertension.

Get Spiritual

A study conducted by the formidably sober and scientific Harvard University found that patients who were prayed for recovered quicker than those who were not, even if they were not aware of the prayer.

9.2. PROSTATE HEALTH

The topic on prostate is misleading. Is prostate strictly for men? Yes, only men have prostate and only men over 40years but the healthcare enlightenment is for everyone. There is no woman who does not know a man 40 years and above – father, uncle, brother, son, friend, neighbor, colleague …

Essentially looking at background on prostate health, everyone has a pair of kidneys. The job of the kidney is to remove waste. It is the waste management company of your body. Every day, your blood passes through the kidney several times to be filtered. As the blood is filtered, urine is formed and stored in a temporary storage tank called the urinary bladder. If there were to be no urinary bladder, as a man walks on the road, urine will be dropping.

Now think of the plumbing work in your house. Think of the urinary bladder as the overhead storage tank. From the storage tank, a good plumber will run pipes to other parts of the house, including the kitchen. God in His wisdom ran pipes from our urinary bladder to the tip of the penis. The pipe is called the urethra. Just below the bladder and surrounding the urethra is a little organ called the prostate gland.

The prostate gland is the size of a walnut and weighs about 20grams. Its job is to make the seminal fluid which is stored in the seminal vesicle. During sexual intercourse, seminal fluid comes down the urethra and mixes with the sperms produced in the testicles to form the semen. So semen technically is not sperm. It is sperm + seminal fluid. The seminal fluid lubricates the sperm.

After age 40, for reasons that may be hormonal, the prostate gland begins to enlarge. From 20 grams it may grow to almost 100 grams. As it enlarges, it squeezes the urethra and the man begins to notice changes in the way he urinate.

If you have a son under 10, and if he has a little mischief like we all did at that age, when he comes out to urinate, he can target the ceiling and the jet will hit target. Call his father to do same, impossible! His urine stream is weak, cannot travel a long distance and sometimes may come straight down on his legs. So he may need to stand in awkward position to urinate.

Not many men will be worried their urine stream cannot hit the ceiling. Toilets are on the floor and not on the ceiling. But other symptoms begin to show.

Terminal dripping

The man begins to notice that after urinating and repacking, urine still drops on his pants. This is the reason why after an older man urinates, he has to ring bell. A younger man simply delivers to the last drop and walks away. Just see an older man coming from the bathroom. Sometimes he may clutch the newspaper closely to hide the urine stains, particularly on plain colored trousers.

Hesitancy

At this point you wait longer for the urine flow to start. There are two (2) valves that must open for you to urinate – the internal and external sphincters. Both open but because of obstructions in the urethra, you wait long for the flow to start.

Incomplete emptying

You have this feeling immediately after urinating that there is still something left. As all these things happen, the bladder begins to work harder to compensate for the obstruction in the urethra. The frequency of urination goes up. Urgency sets in. sometimes you have to practically run into the toilet. Nocturia also becomes common. You wake up more than 2 times at night to urinate. Your wife begins to complain and may not talk to anyone even at this point. Then the more serious complications start.

Stored urine gets infected and there may be burning sensation when urinating. Stored urine forms crystals. Crystals come together to form stone either in the bladder or in the kidney. Stones may block the urethra.

Chronic urinary retention sets in. The bladder stores more and more urine. The size of the bladder is 40 - 60 cl. A bottle of coke is 50cl. As the bladder stores more urine it can enlarge up to 300cl. An overfilled bladder may leak and this leads to wetting/urinary incontinence. Also the volume may put pressure on the kidney and may lead to kidney damage.

What may likely bring the man to hospital is acute urinary retention. He wakes up one day and he is not able to pass urine. Everything I have described above is associated with prostate enlargement, technically called *benign prostate hyperplasia.*

There are other diseases of the prostate like:

- Prostatitis – inflammation of the prostate
- Prostate cancer – cancer of the prostate.

The bad news and good news:

The bad news is that everyman will have prostate enlargement if he lives long enough.

The good news is that there are life style changes that can help the man after (forty) 40 to maintain optimum prostate health.

Nutrition

Look at what you eat. Thirty three percent (33%) of all cancers, according to the US National Cancer Institute is related to what we eat.

Red meat everyday triples your chances of prostate disease. Milk everyday doubles your risk. Not taking fruits/vegetables daily quadruples your risk.

Tomatoes are very good for men. If that is the only thing your wife can present in the evening, eat it with joy. It has loads of lycopene. Lycopene is the most potent natural antioxidant.

Foods that are rich in zinc are also good for men. We recommend pumpkin seeds.

Zinc is about the most essential element for male sexuality and fertility. Men need more zinc than women. Every time a man ejaculates he loses 15mg of zinc. Zinc is also important for alcohol metabolism. Your liver needs zinc to metabolize alcohol.

Alcohol consumption
As men begin to have urinary symptoms associated with prostate enlargement, it is important they look at alcohol consumption. More fluid in means more fluid out. Drink less. Drink slowly.

Exercise
Exercise helps build the muscle tone. Every man should exercise. Men over 40 should avoid high impact exercise like jogging. It puts pressure on the knees. Cycling is bad news for the prostate. Brisk walking is recommended.

Sitting
When we sit, two-third of our weight rests on the pelvic bones. Men who sit longer are more prone to prostate symptoms. Do not sit for long hours. Walk around as often as you can. Sit on comfortable chairs. Divided saddle chair is recommended if you must sit long hours.

Dressing
Men should avoid tight underwear. It impacts circulation around the groin and heats it up a bit. While the physiological temperature is 37 degrees, the groin has an optimal temperature of about 33 degrees. Pant is a no - no for men. Wear boxers. Wear breathable clothing.

Smoking
Avoid smoking. It affects blood vessels and impact circulation around the groin.

Sex
Regular sex is good for the prostate. Celibates are more prone to prostate illness. While celibacy is a moral decision, it is not a biological adaptation. Your prostate gland is designed to empty its contents regularly.

9.3. AGE GRACEFULLY-- TRICKS TO KEEPING YOUR YOUTHFUL GLOW WITH EACH PASSING YEAR

Skip the fancy skincare routine

Cut through the anti-aging aisle. If you use a sunscreen, retinoid, and moisturizer starting at age 20, your skin will look much younger compared to someone who didn't use them," says New York City dermatologist Lance Brown, MD, clinical assistant professor of dermatology at New York University School of Medicine. Applying SPF every morning is a must, along with keeping cells plump and hydrated with moisturizer.

Retinoids are where the magic happens, because the vitamin A derivative essentially teaches your skin to act young again, stimulating the collagen that prevents fine lines.

Embrace change

Embrace change as life is change. Resisting it wastes precious time and energy. Living for it can create adventures you never thought possible.

Exercise regularly

A minimum of 45 minutes of aerobic exercise, three to four times a week, will keep your heart young while improving your figure, mood and brainpower. Whatever your motivation to work out—feeling good, blowing off stress, losing weight—you can add one more to the list: staying young. In a study on older adults, those who exercised, functioned physiologically similar to younger people. So it keeps you young on the inside, but what about the outside? "Your skin is the largest organ in your body and the only one you can see. Anything that is good for your body is good for your skin. While you may have heard warnings that certain workouts (namely running) can cause wrinkles and sagging from the up-and-down motion, that is not the case. Whatever you love doing—whether that is running, spinning, or lifting—keep on doing it.

Eat a mostly Mediterranean diet

Eat lots of fruits and vegetables. Cook with olive oil instead of butter. Eat with friends and family. Prepare food together. Eat the things you like.

Eat smartly. Eat your vitamins: the best way to get vitamins and minerals is from a well-balanced diet.

Value your body
Value your body. If you do, you will participate in less risky behavior that could harm your health. Do not let yourself be diminished by anyone. You are you. No one else is, and that is very important.

Do not cake aging
Aging do not hide behind makeup. If you have wrinkles, brown spots, and bags, you are probably tempted to slap on a thick coat of foundation and powder all over your face. That technique backfires. Makeup cannot completely cover aging and do not cake it on, but rather build it for a youthful, healthy glow.

Embrace technology
The internet can take you places you would never otherwise see or experience. You can learn something new from someone of any age.

Control blood pressure
High blood pressure today sets you up for dementia later. Take control of how you react to things. Little things can really bring you down if you let them. But you do not have to let them.

Learn something new every day
The more you challenge your brain, the better it performs, studies suggest. Better to learn varied things, and participate in group activities.

Face and hands aging care
Your face and hands are two body parts that get the most sun. But since you are busy slathering on moisturizers and anti-aging products on your face, your complexion may look young while your hands betray that with brown spots and wrinkles. The same exact products

you use for your face can go on your hands. So when you use a retinoid at night, rub a small amount to the backs of your hands. After slathering on a good SPF moisturizer in the morning, do the same for your hands.

Take care of mental health
Middle age is time to get rid of emotional baggage that stresses you out. Cut down or eliminate multi-tasking. Research shows people do not do it very well, and it often just causes undue stress. If you are depressed, seek professional help. There are solutions.

Confidence aging
Women who age gracefully have something big in common: confidence, they exude confidence. Do not do anything with the idea that you are trying to look younger—that can cause big missteps in your sense of style and how you maintain your beauty routine. Make your goal to be the best you can look, it can pay off down the line: In an earlier study from Yale University, people who had more positive beliefs about aging lived 7.5 years longer than those with more downtrodden.

Style aging- everyday habits that age you
Have you avoided changing your style since you got your first job? A lot of women struggle to get out of a style rut and run the risk of looking like they are stuck in a time warp. Finding a new style that works for your life today. The right cut can pay off in other ways.

Avoid diabetes
Uncontrolled diabetes can thin the brain's cortex, increasing risk of Alzheimer's and other forms of dementia. Again, diet and exercise are the best prevention.

Trends aging
Being a certain age does not mean you have to change into an "older" style. Women who age gracefully do not step aside from

trends because of their age. Dress in current styles. By adding a trendy piece to a classic outfit, you will look and feel good. Up on the latest trends gives your look that extra secret sauce. It is a great instant energy booster; not to mention, a bonus to your confidence and self-esteem.

Share happiness
Make a point to spread joy whenever possible. It feels good to make someone else feel good, and it's very inexpensive to do. Laugh and cry. But laugh a lot more. It feels good by releasing endorphins – the body's natural feel-good chemicals.

Embrace gray hair
Those who age gracefully are not afraid to embrace their grays. Men and Women can look stunning when they go gray. You may need a super sharp sophisticated cut to really show it off. Maintain your vibrant hue with a blue-violet based shampoo, which prevents yellowing from minerals in the water,

Take adequate sleep
It is not called beauty sleep for nothing. Poor quality sleep not only increases the visible signs of aging around your face, but also makes you feel less attractive. Sleep helps your skin naturally ward off the damaging effects of the sun, slowing down the aging process.

Travel
Whether it is a trip to the shopping mall, theater, a sports or social event, or even a different state or country, little and big adventures can produce wonderful results and memories.

Get a yearly medical check-up
Get a yearly medical check-up. While it is no guarantee you will live longer, it can help you catch health issues early and fend off other potential health problems or challenges.

9.4. HEALTH BENEFITS OF ENVIRONMENTAL SANITATION

Environmental sanitation is very vital for everyone and in order to live a world free from diseases, we must task ourselves in a more collaborative and more sustained ways to frequently embark on general cleaning exercises in our houses, homes and our communities. Health experts have indicated that clean environment initiative has drastically reduced the burden of malarial diseases and other health related issues.

Sanitation is the hygienic means of promoting health through prevention of human contact with the hazards of wastes as well as the treatment and proper disposal of sewage wastewater. Hazards can be either physical, microbiological, biological or chemical agents of disease. Wastes that can cause health problems include human and animal feces, solid wastes, domestic wastewater (sewage, sullage, greywater), industrial wastes and agricultural wastes.

- Environmental sanitation keeps away diseases causing organism (pathogens) from our environment.
- Improved sanitation leads to a reduction in diarrheal morbidity and other related maternal health issues.
- Improved drainage and solid waste management reduce breeding grounds for mosquitoes, and improved sanitation and hygiene for people with HIV and AIDS help prevent health complications.
- Improved excreta disposal, solid waste management and drainage protects the quality of water resources and creates a clean and safe environment for healthy living.

CHAPTER 10

DISEASES, CAUSES, SYMPTOMS AND PREVENTIVE TREATMENTS

DISEASE IS DEFINED by Farlex Partner Medical Dictionary as any deviation from or interruption of the normal structure or function of any body part, organ, or system that is manifested by a characteristic set of symptoms and signs and whose etiology, pathology, and prognosis may be known or unknown.

The risk of illness is very real, and people need to be aware of diseases that may be present and how to avoid these diseases.

This brief listing of some of the most notorious diseases explains their causes, symptoms, prevention and treatment.

Diseases	Causes	Symptoms	Prevention/Home Treatment	Warning Signals (See Doctor)
Acute upper respiratory tract infections		Common cold and fever Heavy coughing Chest pain and pain between shoulder blades in pneumonia	Prevent overcrowding in confined spaces	
Bird flu also known as Avian flu or influenza	Caused by viruses that infect birds and make them ill. It is an infectious disease of birds caused by type A strains of the influenza virus.	Symptoms in humans can vary and range from "typical" flu symptoms (fever, sore throat, muscle pain) to eye infections and pneumonia. The disease caused by the H5N1 virus is a particularly severe form of pneumonia that leads to viral pneumonia and multiorgan failure in many people who become infected.	Avoid sources of exposure whenever possible. Adequate hand hygiene. People who work with poultry or who respond to avian influenza outbreaks are advised to follow recommended biosecurity and infection control practices. Antiviral drugs can be used to treat illness.	**Immediate field investigation of every possible case to confirm the diagnosis, identify the source, and determine whether human-to-human transmission is occurring.** **See doctor immediately after detection or diagnosis.**
Cholera	When bacteria excreted in faeces comes into contact with drinking water	Watery diarrhea, which is pale and flaky and looks like rice water. High fluid loss may be as high as 1 litre every hour	Only drink boiled water or water that has been sterilized or treated in another way	**If the fluid loss is not replaced and exceeds 5-10 litres, it can be fatal** **Extensive dehydration**

	Spread to food if people do not wash their hands thoroughly after using the toilet		Boil unpasteurised milk before you drink it	
			Properly prepare food and serve when still hot. If it is allowed to stand at room temperature for several hours other bacteria may develop	
	Spread through fish and shellfish from contaminated water		Avoid raw fish and shellfish	
			Avoid raw fruit and vegetables, unless you peel it yourself	
			Consume large quantities of fluid with salt and sugar.	
			Take ORS Salts with zinc tablets.	
			You can prepare the mix by mixing boiled and cooled/clean water 1 litre (5 cups) + ½ level tea spoon salt + 2 level tea spoon sugar + lemon juice (optional). Stir vigorously.	
Diarrhea	Bacterial and viral infections	Frequent, watery motions	Drink more fluids (3-4 litres a day); preferably containing sugar and salts.	**Blood in the motions**
				Pus in the motions
	Food poisoning	Nausea, vomiting	Eat something containing salt	**(yellow mucus)**

	Transmitted from person to person	Fever	Avoid foods containing milk for a couple of days after recovery	**Inability to drink liquids because of vomiting**
		Dehydration		
			Eat vegetables that have been boiled or peeled	**Dehydration-symptoms include excreting small**
			People with inflammation or sores on their hands should	**amounts of dark urine, drowsiness, dry mucous**
			not prepare food	**membranes and thirst**
				Pronounced drowsiness
				Acute diarrhea in infants or old people
				Diarrhea has lasted more than one to two weeks
Dengue and Dengue Hemorrhagic Fever (DHF)		High fever	Same as malaria (See malaria)	**Same as malaria (See malaria)**
		Head ache	Items that are used to store water in houses should be covered	
		Pain in muscles and joints		
		Red spots on Skin		

Diphtheria	Bacterial disease By coughing or sneezing	Respiratory diphtheria causes a sore throat and fever, and sometimes swelling of the neck. In severe cases it can cause a membrane to form over the throat, which results in breathing problems. Cutaneous diphtheria affects the skin, causing infected lesions to form.	Treated by hospitalization and antibiotics Vaccination	**Diphtheria can lead to coma and death if it goes untreated.**
Ebola virus disease (EVD)	Rare and often-fatal infection caused by one of the five strains of the Ebola virus: Ebola virus (Zaire ebolavirus); Sudan virus (Sudan ebolavirus); Taï Forest virus (Taï Forest ebolavirus, formerly Côte d'Ivoire ebolavirus); and Bundibugyo virus (Bundibugyo ebolavirus).	A fever greater than 101.5 degrees Fahrenheit (38.6 degrees Celsius) Muscle pain or aches Severe headache Weakness Bloody diarrhea Vomiting Abdominal pain	There is no cure for Ebola, though researchers are working on it. Treatment includes an experimental serum that destroys infected cells. Doctors manage the symptoms of Ebola with: Fluids and electrolytes Oxygen Blood pressure medication Blood transfusions Treatment for other infections	**See Doctor or physician immediately you observe the symptoms. Ebola virus kills fast.**

Hepatitis A, B C, D and E	Viral hepatitis, including hepatitis A, hepatitis B, hepatitis C, hepatitis D and hepatitis E, are distinct diseases that affect the liver and have different hepatitis symptoms and treatments.	Loss of appetite	Hepatitis A	Always check with your doctor if you have any of the signs of hepatitis.
		Fatigue	Immunization of children (1-18 years of age).	
		Mild fever	Adults need a booster dose six to 12 months following the initial dose of vaccine. The vaccine is thought to be effective for 15–20 years or more.	If you do not get treatment, it can lead to cirrhosis, a serious scarring of your liver.
		Muscle or joint aches		
		Nausea and vomiting	In General:	
	Other causes of hepatitis include recreational drugs and prescription medications.	Pain in your belly	Wash your hands after going to the bathroom and before fixing food or eating.	
		Some people have other issues, such as:	Use latex condoms, which may lower the risk of transmission.	
		Dark urine		
	Hepatitis type is determined by laboratory tests.	Light-colored stools	Avoid tap water when traveling to certain countries or regions.	
		Jaundice (yellowing of the skin and whites of the eyes)	Do not share drug needles.	
		Itchy feeling	Do not share personal items—such as toothbrushes, razors and nail clippers—with an infected person.	
		Mental changes, such as stupor (being in a daze) or coma	Bed rest, abstaining from alcohol, and taking medication to help relieve symptoms.	
		Bleeding inside your body	Most people who have hepatitis A and E get well on	

		their own after a few weeks.		
HIV/AIDS	Anal or vaginal sexual intercourse and illicit injectable drug use commonly transmit HIV. Infected mothers may also transmit HIV to their child during pregnancy or breastfeeding. Less common routes of transmission include needle-stick injuries or exposure to contaminated blood.	Rapid weight loss. Recurring fever or profuse night sweats. Extreme and unexplained tiredness. Prolonged swelling of the lymph glands in the armpits, groin, or neck. Diarrhea that lasts for more than a week. Sores of the mouth, anus, or genitals. Pneumonia.	There is no vaccine to prevent HIV infection and no cure for AIDS. But it is possible to protect yourself and others from infection. That means educating yourself about HIV and avoiding any behavior that allows HIV-infected fluids — blood, semen, vaginal secretions and breast milk — into your body. Treatment with highly active antiretroviral therapy (HAART or ART) dramatically increases life expectancy although it does not cure HIV infection.	**See Doctor when tested positive to HIV to confirm the diagnosis and discuss possible treatment and prevention regimen.**
Influenza or "flu"	Contagious virus	Body aches, sore throat, headache, fever, coughing, and chills	Treated by antiviral medicines Seasonal vaccination	**The disease can be fatal; especially for babies, the elderly, and people with weakened immune systems**
Malaria	Anopheles mosquito biting a person who has malaria parasites in their blood	Fever and shivering. The attack begins with fever, with the temperature rising as high as 40°C and falling again over a period of several hours Painful muscles	Prevent stagnation of water Spray insecticides and larvicidal agents on stagnant water pools	**May become fatal unless medical care is provided within first 48 hours.**

		and joints	Applying mosquito repellents on exposed skin	
		Diarrhea, nausea and vomiting	Using mosquito nets	
			Wear clothes that leave very little skin exposed	
			By taking anti-malaria drugs	
Measles	A highly contagious disease caused by a virus	Early symptoms include fever, cough, red eyes, and a runny nose. During the first few days, the characteristic measles rash appears, beginning with white spots in the mouth and spreading to a red rash that covers the entire body	There is no specific remedy available for measles, so treatment usually consists of bed rest and easing symptoms Immunization	**Severe cases of measles can cause diarrhea, ear infection, pneumonia, encephalitis (swelling of the brain), and death**
Mumps	A contagious viral disease	Causes painful swelling of the salivary glands "Chipmunk cheeks." Fever, headache, sore muscles, and fatigue	Avoid contact with the respiratory secretions of an infected person Immunization- Mumps vaccination	**Serious complications are rare, and may include encephalitis (swelling of the brain), inflammation of the sex organs, and deafness**
Poliomyelitis or Polio	Viral infection spread by person-to-person contact	Symptoms vary according to the type of infection, and three basic patterns are common:	Treatments vary according to the form of the disease, and may include antibiotics, pain-relieving medication, and physical therapy to strengthen weak muscles	**In Paralytic-poliomyelitis, muscle weakness comes on quickly and progresses to Paralysis**

		Subclinical-symptoms may include fatigue, headache, sore throat, mild fever, and vomiting	Immunization of children	
		Nonparalytic-poliomyelitis. Symptoms may		
		include back pain, neck pain, fatigue, diarrhea, headache, leg pain, fever, muscle stiffness, painful rash, and vomiting		
		Paralytic- poliomyelitis (the most serious kind of		
		Polio infection.) Symptoms may include fever, breathing difficulty, constipation, headache,		
		muscle pain, muscle spasms, and muscle		
		weakness on one side of the body		
Typhoid	Salmonella typhi bacteria	The patient's temperature rises gradually to 40°C	Same as for Diarrhea	**See a Doctor or Physician**
	Contaminated food or water		Proper hygiene and sanitation, but vaccines against the disease are also available	
	Improper hand-washing and poor sanitation	Bouts of sweating, no appetite, coughing and headache		
		Constipation and skin symptoms		
		Increasing listlessness and clouding of consciousness		

10.1. RISKS POSED BY CORPSES

Workers who routinely handle corpses may have a risk of contracting tuberculosis, blood borne viruses (such as Hepatitis B/C and HIV), and gastrointestinal infections (such as diarrhea, typhoid/paratyphoid fevers, hepatitis A, cholera and others).

- Exposure to blood borne viruses occurs due to direct contact with non-intact skin of blood or body fluid, injury from bone fragments and needles, or exposure to the mucous membranes from splashing of blood or body fluid.
- Gastrointestinal infections are more common as dead bodies commonly leak faeces.

Transmission occurs via the faeco-oral route through direct contact with the body and soiled clothes or contaminated vehicles or equipment. Dead bodies contaminating the water supply may also cause gastrointestinal infections.

The public and emergency workers alike should avoid panic and inappropriate disposal of bodies, and to take adequate precautions in handling the dead.

10.2. PREVENTIVE MEASURES FOR WORKERS THAT ROUTINELY HANDLE CORPSES

- Graveyards should be at least 30m from groundwater sources used for drinking water
- The bottom of any grave must be at least 1.5m above the water table with a 0.7m unsaturated zone. Surface water from graveyards must not enter inhabited areas
- Ensure use of gloves, masks and eyewear- protection to reduce the risk of exposure to blood and body fluids
- Ensure use and correct disposal of gloves and masks etc. (no re-use)

- Ensure use of body bags
- Ensure hand-washing with soap after handling bodies and before eating
- Ensure disinfection of vehicles and equipment.
- Bodies do not need to be disinfected before disposal (except in case of cholera)
- Vaccinate workers against hepatitis B.

GLOSSARY

Abscess: an abscess is a tender, easily pressed mass generally surrounded by a coloured area from pink to deep red. The middle of an abscess is full of pus and debris.

Abuse: improper or excessive use or treatment of something.

Acne: acne vulgaris (or simply acne) is a long-term skin condition characterized by areas of blackheads, whiteheads, pimples, greasy skin, and possibly scarring.

Addiction: a physical and/or psychological need for a substance, due to regular, continued use.

Additive: A substance added in small amounts to something else to improve, strengthen, or otherwise alter it.

Alcoholic beverage: is a drink that typically contains 3%-40% alcohol (ethanol).

Alcoholism: an addiction to the consumption of alcoholic liquor or the mental illness and compulsive behavior resulting from alcohol dependency.

Algae: Algae are photosynthetic organisms that occur in most habitats. They vary from small, single-celled forms to complex multicellular forms, such as the giant kelps that grow to 65 meters in length.

Amenorrhea: Amenorrhea is the medical term for the absence of menstrual periods, either on a permanent or temporary basis. Amenorrhea can be classified as primary or secondary.

Anandamide: a derivative of arachidonic acid that occurs naturally in the brain and in some foods (as chocolate) and that binds to the same brainreceptors as the cannabinoids (as THC).

Anhydrase: An enzyme that catalyzes the removal of water from a material or compound.

Anxiolytics: a medication or other intervention that inhibits anxiety.

Artery: A blood vessel that carries oxygen-rich blood from the heart to the body.

Atherosclerosis: Built up of fat or cholesterol deposits inside the artery wall, causing narrowing of the arteries.

Atrophy: is the weakening, loss, wasting away, break-down or growth-halt of something such as a body part.

Azeotrope: a liquid mixture of two or more substances that boils at a constant characteristic temperature lower or higher than any of its components and that retains the same composition in the vapor state as in the liquid state.

Bajra: (In South Asia) pearl millet or similar grain.

Barbiturate: a strong drug that makes people calm or helps them to sleep.

Bout: a short period of intense activity of a specified kind or an attack of illness or strong emotion.

Brisk: active, fast, and energetic.

Bristle: a short stiff hair, typically one of those on an animal's skin, a man's face, or a plant.

Calorie: a unit used in measuring the amount of energy, food provides when eaten and digested.

Cardiac arrhythmias: an arrhythmia is an irregular heartbeat - the heart may beat too fast (tachycardia), too slowly (bradycardia), too early (premature contraction) or too irregularly (fibrillation).

Carpopedal spasm: a spasmodic contraction of the muscles of the hands and feet or especially of the wrists and ankles in disorders such as alkalosis and tetany.

Casseroles: a large, deep dish used both in the oven and as a serving vessel. The word is also used for the food cooked and served in such a vessel, with the cookware itself called a casserole dish or casserole pan. Food such as a stew.

Cathartic: providing psychological relief through the open expression of strong emotions; causing catharsis

Cessation: Cessation is an end to something, such as the stopping of a bad habit, like the cessation of smoking.

Chapatti: an unleavened flatbread (also known as roti) from Sri Lanka, India, Nepal, Bangladesh and Pakistan. It is a common staple in South Asia as well as amongst South Asian expatriates throughout the world.

Cholesterol: cholesterol is a fatty substance found in the bloodstream and in all the cells in your body.

Cinnamic acid: It is a white crystalline compound that is slightly soluble in water, and freely soluble in many organic solvents.

Cognitive: of, relating to, or involving conscious mental activities (such as thinking, understanding, learning, and remembering).

Comorbid: two disorders or illnesses occur in the same person, simultaneously or sequentially.

Constipation: a condition in which there is difficulty in emptying the bowels, usually associated with hardened feces.

Cytochrome: any of several intracellular hemoprotein respiratory pigments that are enzymes functioning in electron transport as carriers of electrons.

Dehydrogenase: an enzyme that accelerates the removal of hydrogen from metabolites and its transfer to other substances.

Dementia: is a general term for a decline in mental ability severe enough to interfere with daily life. Memory loss is an example.

Dermabrasion: sanding the skin with a wire brush to remove the epidermis and dermis.

Dessert: a usually sweet course or dish, as of fruit, ice cream, or pastry, served at the end of a meal.

Diabetes: A disease in which either the body does not produce enough insulin or the body's cells do not effectively use the insulin produced.

Diabetic retinopathy: also known as diabetic eye disease is when damage occurs to the retina due to diabetes.

Diet: a particular selection of food, especially as designed or prescribed to improve a person's physical condition or to prevent or treat a disease.

Digesta: something undergoing digestion (as food in the stomach).

Disorder: a derangement or abnormality of function; a morbid physical or mental state.

Dopamine: dopamine is a neurotransmitter. It is a chemical messenger that helps in the transmission of signals in the brain and other vital areas.

Dyspepsia: dyspepsia, also known as indigestion or upset stomach, is a term that describes discomfort or pain in the upper abdomen.

Earache: pain inside the ear.

Elastin: the fibers that give your skin strength and elasticity.

Elation: a feeling or state of great joy or pride; exultant gladness; high spirits.

Emollient: non-cosmetic moisturizers which come in the form of creams, ointments, lotions and gels.

Emulsifier: a substance that stabilizes an emulsion, in particular a food additive used to stabilize processed foods.

Endorphins: are among the brain chemicals known as neurotransmitters, which function to transmit electrical signals within the nervous system.

Entrée: a small dish served before the main course of a meal, or the main dish of a meal.

Ester: a compound produced by the reaction between an acid and an alcohol with the elimination of a molecule of water.

Etiology: the study of causation, or origination.

Euphoria: a feeling of great happiness or well-being, commonly exaggerated and not necessarily well founded.

Excipient: a natural or synthetic substance formulated alongside the active ingredient of a medication, included for the purpose of bulking up formulations that contain potent active ingredients.

Exercise: activity requiring physical effort, carried out especially to sustain or improve health and fitness.

Fad: something that people are interested in for a short period of time.

Faeco-oral: a passage or transfer, as of a disease from one individual to another.

Filling: a way to restore a tooth damaged by decay back to its normal function and shape.

Floss: clean between (one's teeth) with dental floss.

Fracture: the breaking of a bone, cartilage, or the like, or the resulting condition.

Gene: the basic physical and functional unit of heredity.

Glaucoma: disease that damages your eye's optic nerve. It usually happens when fluid builds up in the front part of your eye.

Glycemic index (GI): or glycaemic index (GI) is a number associated with a particular type of food that indicates the food's effect on a person's blood glucose (also called blood sugar) level. A value of 100 represents the standard, an equivalent amount of pure glucose.

Goiter: is an abnormal enlargement of your thyroid gland. Your thyroid is a butterfly-shaped gland located at the base of your neck just below your Adam's apple.

Goose bumps: **goose pimples** or **goose** flesh, the medical term cutis anserina or horripilation, are the bumps on a person's skin at the base of body hairs which may involuntarily develop when a person is cold or experiences strong emotions such as fear, nostalgia, pleasure, euphoria, awe, admiration, and sexual arousal.

Gum: the firm area of pink flesh around the roots of the teeth in the upper or lower jaw.

Halitosis: an unpleasant odor from the mouth, commonly referred to as **bad breath**. Halitosis can be caused by the consumption of certain foods, poor oral hygiene, alcohol or tobacco use, dry mouth, or by certain chronic medical conditions.

Hallucination: a sensory experience of something that does not exist outside the mind, caused by various physical and mental disorders, or by reaction to certain toxic substances, and usually manifested as visual or auditory images.

Hepatitis: inflammation of the liver, caused by a virus or a toxin and characterized by jaundice, liver enlargement, and fever.

HIV: Human immunodeficiency virus is a virus that attacks the immune system, the body's natural defense system. Without a strong immune system, the body has trouble fighting off disease. Both the virus and the infection it causes are called HIV.

Humectants: a substance, especially a skin lotion or a food additive, used to reduce the loss of moisture.

Hyper: a prefix appearing in loanwords from Greek, where it meant "over," "beyond" or "above", usually implying excess or exaggeration (hyperbole).

Hypernatremia: a common electrolyte problem and is defined as a rise in serum sodium concentration to a value exceeding 145 mmol/L. The normal adult value for sodium is 136-145 mEq/L.

Hyperthermia: the condition of having a body temperature greatly above normal.

Hypertrichosis: a skin abnormality that results in excessive growth of hair. It can be localized to one part of the body, or affect in full. It can affect men or women and is mostly secondary to a genetic disease that causes a hormonal disorder.

Hypo: a prefix that means "beneath" or "below," as in hypodermic, below the skin. It also means "less than normal," especially in medical terms like hypoglycemia.

Hypokalemia: refers to a lower than normal potassium level in your bloodstream.

Hypomanic: an abnormality of mood resembling mania (persistent elevated or expansive mood, hyperactivity, inflated self-esteem, and so on) but of lesser intensity.

Hyponatremia: excess water intake, without replenishment of sodium and potassium salts, leads to hyponatremia.

Hypotension: low blood pressure. However, for many people, low blood pressure can cause symptoms of dizziness and fainting. In severe cases, low blood pressure can be life-threatening

Hypothyroidism: also known as underactive thyroid, is a condition where the thyroid gland does not create enough of a thyroid hormone called thyroxine. It results in retardation of growth and mental development in children and adults.

Hypoxia: a condition in which the body or a region of the body is deprived of adequate oxygen supply.

Immune system: the bodily system that protects the body from foreign substances, cells, and tissues by producing the immune response and that includes especially the thymus, spleen, lymph nodes, special deposits of lymphoid tissue (as in the gastrointestinal tract and bone marrow), lymphocytes including the B cells and T cells.

Insomnia: is a persistent disorder that can make it hard to fall asleep, hard to stay asleep or both, despite the opportunity for adequate sleep.

Intranasal: lying within or administered by way of the nasal structures.

Irritability: the ability of the cell to receive and respond to a stimulus.

Jain: An ascetic religion of India, founded in the sixth century (Before Christ, BC), that teaches the immortality and transmigration of the soul and denies the existence of a supreme being.

Laryngospasm: an uncontrolled/involuntary muscular contraction (spasm) of the vocal folds. The condition typically lasts less than 60 seconds, and causes a partial blocking of breathing in, while breathing out remains easier.

Leeks: a vegetable that has long green leaves rising from a thick white base and that tastes like a mild onion.

Lipid: a fat-like molecule that does not have the ability to dissolve in water and includes molecules such as cholesterol and triglycerides. Lipids are one of the major building blocks of animal cells. Many times, lipids will be referred to as a "fat".

Lipoid: an oily organic compound insoluble in water but soluble in organic solvents; essential structural component of living cells (along with proteins and carbohydrates). Any of various substances, such as lecithin, that resemble fat.

Lycopene: a red pigment found predominantly in tomatoes (and also in some other fruits) that gives them their color. Lycopene has antioxidant properties and has been claimed to "promote a healthy heart" and to reduce the risk of cancer.

Lymph gland: one of many small organs in the body that produce the white blood cells needed for the body to fight infection.

Lymphatic: small thin channels similar to blood vessels that do not carry blood, but collect and carry tissue fluid (called lymph) from the body to ultimately drain back into the blood stream.

Macromineral: inorganic nutrients needed in relatively high daily amounts (that is, more than 100 mg per day), for example, calcium, phosphorus, sodium.

Macular degeneration: is the leading cause of severe vision loss in people over age 60. It occurs when the small central portion of the retina, known as the **macula**, deteriorates. The retina is the light-sensing nerve tissue at the back of the eye.

Mania: an abnormally elevated mood state characterized by such symptoms as inappropriate elation, increased irritability, severe insomnia, grandiose notions, increased speed and/or volume of speech, disconnected and racing thoughts, increased sexual desire, markedly increased energy and activity level, poor judgment, and inappropriate social behavior. A mild form in mania that does not require hospitalization is termed hypomania. Mania that also features symptoms of depression ("agitated depression") is called mixed mania.

Marathon: a footrace run on an open course usually of 26 miles, 385 yards (42.2 kilometers); broadly: a long-distance race.

Matrix model: is an intensive outpatient treatment approach for stimulant abuse and dependence that was developed through 20 years of experience in real-world treatment settings.

Micromineral: a mineral of which only trace amounts are needed in the diet.

Misuse: to use (something) in the wrong way or for the wrong purpose.

Morbidity: the incidence of disease (the rate of sickness).

Myelin: the fatty substance that covers and protects nerves.

Myelinization: the formation of the myelin sheath around a nerve fiber. Also known as myelination.

Myokines: are proteins secreted from skeletal muscle that can execute important biological functions locally in the muscle (paracrine) or in other organs like the brain, heart and pancreas (endocrine).

Neural: relating to, or affecting a nerve or the nervous system.

Neurobics: tasks which activate the brain's own biochemical pathways and to bring new pathways online that can help to strengthen or preserve brain circuits.

Neuron: a cell that carries messages between the brain and other parts of the body and that is the basic unit of the nervous system.

Neurotoxin: a substance that can damage or destroy the nervous system.

Neurotransmitters: chemicals that relay signals from neuron to neuron.

Nutrition: the process of taking in food and using it for growth, metabolism, and repair.

Occlusive: serving to close; denoting a bandage or dressing that closes a wound and excludes it from the air.

Ocular hypertension: is an eye pressure of greater than 21 mm Hg. Normal eye pressure ranges from 10-21 mm Hg.

Oligosaccharides: a carbohydrate consisting of a relatively small and specifiable number of monosaccharides joined together. Lactose, maltose, and sucrose are oligosaccharides consisting of two simple sugars.

Osteoporosis: a medical condition in which the bones become brittle and fragile from loss of tissue, typically as a result of hormonal changes, or deficiency of calcium or vitamin D.

Ounce: a unit of weight equal to 437.5 grains or 1/16 pound (28.35 grams) avoirdupois. One ounce weighs about the same as a slice of bread. Abbreviation: oz.

Oxidase: any of various enzymes that catalyze oxidations; especially: one able to react directly with molecular oxygen.

Ozone layer: the layer of air around the earth that helps to regulate the temperature.

Palpitation: a sensation in which a person is aware of an irregular, hard, or rapid heartbeat.

Pancreatitis: sudden inflammation of the pancreas.

Pap smear: also called a **Pap test**, is a procedure to test for cervical cancer in women.

Paranoia: is being suspicious, having illusions about being followed or persecuted, or about being afraid or distrustful of others.

Pathology: a branch of medical science that studies the nature, effects, causes and consequences of disease.

Pellagra: a disease due to deficiency of niacin, a B-complex vitamin. It is characterized by dermatitis, diarrhoea, and mental disturbance, and is often linked to over-dependence on maize as a staple food.

Phytochemicals: non-nutritive plant chemicals that have protective or disease preventive properties.

Prognosis: a forecasting of the probable course and outcome of a disease, especially of the chances of recovery.

Psoralen: any of a group of chemical compounds found in certain plants, used to treat psoriasis and vitiligo.

Psoriasis: a common skin condition that changes the life cycle of skin cells. Psoriasis causes cells to build up rapidly on the surface of the skin.

Psychomotor: relating to the origination of movement in conscious mental activity. Examples include driving a car, throwing a ball, and playing a musical instrument.

Psychosis: a symptom or feature of mental illness typically characterized by radical changes in personality, impaired functioning, and a distorted or nonexistent sense of objective reality. In the general sense, a mental illness that markedly interferes with a person's capacity to meet life's everyday demands.

Quercetin: a flavonol found in many fruits, vegetables, leaves and grains. It can be used as an ingredient in supplements, beverages, or foods to reduce allergic responses or boost immunity.

Ragi: Finger millet or Eleusine coracana is an annual plant widely grown as a cereal in the arid areas of Africa and Asia.

Receptor: an organ or cell able to respond to light, heat, or other external stimulus and transmit a signal to a sensory nerve.

Recipes: a set of instructions for preparing a particular dish, including a list of the ingredients required.

Redox: a chemical reaction between two substances in which one substance is oxidized and the other reduced.

Relapse: the return of a disease or health challenge weeks or months after its apparent cessation.

Resentment: a feeling of anger or displeasure about someone or something unfair.

Rhabdomyolysis: the breakdown of muscle tissue that leads to the release of muscle fiber contents into the blood. These substances are harmful to the kidney and often cause kidney damage.

Sake: a wine made from rice.

Salabrasion: using a salt solution to soak the tattooed skin.

Scarification: removing the tattoo with an acid solution and creating a scar in its place.

Schizophreniform: a mental disorder diagnosed when symptoms of **schizophrenia** are present for a significant portion of the time within a one-month period, but signs of disruption are not present for the full six months required for the diagnosis of schizophrenia.

Serotonin: a neurotransmitter that is involved in the transmission of nerve impulses.

Spasms: a sudden uncontrolled and often painful tightening of a muscle.

Sphincter: a ring of muscle surrounding and serving to guard or close an opening or tube, such as the anus or the openings of the stomach.

Spina bifida: a type of birth defect called a neural tube defect. It occurs when the bones of the spine (vertebrae) do not form properly around part of the baby's **spinal** cord.

Steatohepatitis: fatty liver characterized by inflammation of the liver with concurrent fat accumulation in liver.

Stressor: a chemical or biological agent, environmental condition, external stimulus or an event that causes stress to an organism.

Striae distensae: Stretch marks (striae) are pink, red or purple indented streaks that often appear on the abdomen, breasts, upper arms, buttocks and thighs and eventually fade to white or gray. Stretch marks are particularly common in pregnant women, especially during the latter half of pregnancy.

Stroke: the sudden loss of neurologic function due to brain ischaemia or haemorrhage, causing damage or death of brain tissue, also called a cerebrovascular accident or CVA.

Sullage: waste water from household sinks, showers, and baths, but not waste liquid or excreta from toilets.

Sunscreen: a cream or lotion rubbed on to the skin to protect it from the sun. An active ingredient of creams and lotions intended to protect skin from the sun.

Surfactants: compounds that lower the surface tension (or interfacial tension) between two liquids or between a liquid and a solid. Surfactants may act as detergents, wetting agents, emulsifiers, foaming agents, and dispersants.

Tachychardia: also called tachyarrhythmia, is a heart rate that exceeds the normal resting rate (an abnormally rapid heart rate). In general, a resting heart rate over 100 beats per minute (BPM) is accepted as **tachycardia** in adults.

Tactile: of or connected with the sense of touch.

Tattoo: a permanent ink design in the skin applied by needles or a temporary dyed design on the skin.

Tetany: a condition that is due usually to low blood calcium (hypocalcemia) and is characterized by spasms of the hands and feet, cramps, spasm of the voice box (larynx), and overactive neurological reflexes.

Thermometer: an instrument for measuring temperature, especially one having a graduated glass tube with a bulb containing a liquid, typically mercury or colored alcohol, that expands and rises in the tube as the temperature increases

Throb: to beat with increased force or rapidity, as the heart under the influence of emotion or excitement; palpitate.

Throe: a severe pang or spasm of pain, as in childbirth.

Tolerance: the capacity to endure continued subjection to something such as a drug or environmental conditions without adverse reaction.

Topical: something applied to the surface of the body.

Trampoline: a strong fabric sheet connected by springs to a frame, used as a springboard and landing area in doing acrobatic or gymnastic exercises

Tremor: an involuntary shaking of the body or limbs, as from disease, fear, weakness, or excitement; a fit of trembling.

Triglycerides: the major form of fat stored by the body. A **triglyceride** consists of three molecules of fatty acid combined with a molecule of the alcohol glycerol.

Tryptamine: a class of indole alkaloid drugs/chemicals, many of which are psychoactive. Tryptamine are typically serotonin-affecting psychedelics/hallucinogens.

Vasodilation: widening of blood vessels that results from relaxation of the muscular walls of the vessels.

Veggie pantheon: a group of vegetarians.

Veggie: Vegetarian or suitable for vegetarian.

Xerophthalmia: abnormal and prolonged dryness that leads to non-production of tears which helps in lubricating the eyes, typically associated with vitamin A deficiency.

ACRONYMS

ACV: Apple cider vinegar
BD: Bipolar disorder
CBT: Cognitive behavioral therapy
CD: Cyclothymic disorder
DD: Dysthymic disorder
DSM: Diagnostic and Statistical Manual
DV: Diurnal variation of depressive symptoms
ECT: Electroconvulsive therapy
ER: Emergency room
FDA: Food and Drug Administration
GI: Glycemic index
HDL: High-density lipoprotein
HIV: Human immunodeficiency virus
HRT: Hormone replacement therapy
ICD: Implantable cardioverter defibrillator
IPT: Interpersonal therapy or psychodynamic psychotherapy
LSD: Lysergic acid diethylamide
MDD: Major depressive disorder
MDMA: Methylenedioxyphenethylamine
MET: Metabolic Equivalent of Task
MTF: Modulation Transfer Function
NIDA: National Institute on Drug Abuse
ORS: Oral rehydration salts
OTC: Over-the-counter
PCP: Phencyclidine
RDA: Recommended dietary allowances
SAD: Seasonal affective disorder
SPF: Sunscreen Protection Factor
SSRI: Selective serotonin reuptake inhibitor
THC: Tetrahydrocannabinol

TR: Tricuspid regurgitation
URTI: Upper respiratory tract infections
USDA: United States Department of Agriculture
UVR: Ultraviolet radiation